THE NATIONAL CHILDBIRTH TRUST
· · · · · ·
Get Into Shape
After Childbirth
· · · · · ·

THE NATIONAL CHILDBIRTH TRUST
· · · · · ·

Get Into Shape After Childbirth

· · · · · ·

Gillian Fletcher

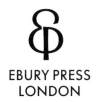

EBURY PRESS
LONDON

First published 1991 by Ebury Press
an imprint of the Random Century Group
Random Century House
20 Vauxhall Bridge Road
London SW1V 2SA

Editor: Felicity Jackson
Designer: Bridgewater Design
Photography Co-ordination: Lynn Sheffield
Illustrations: Helen Chown
Clothes on cover: courtesy of
the Pineapple Dance Centre, London,
and Frocks Away and Early Clothing,
79–85 Fortis Green Road, Muswell Hill, London

British Library Cataloguing in Publication Data

Fletcher, Gillian
National Childbirth Trust: get into shape after
childbirth: a new mother's guide.
I. Title
613.7

ISBN 0-85223-988-2

Typeset in Futura light by Tek Art Limited,
Croydon, Surrey
Printed and bound in Great Britain at
the Bath Press, Avon

CONTENTS

PREFACE

Over the past eighteen years, as a National Childbirth Trust (NCT) antenatal teacher and an obstetric physiotherapist, I have had the privilege of being teacher and confidante to about a thousand women at a most exciting and challenging time in their lives. My main aim has always been to offer them information to enable them to make appropriate choices relating to the experiences before and after birth and to be there to listen and share some of the joy and laughter, disappointment, pain and sorrow. I owe them all a great deal because through my contact with these women and their partners and babies, I have learnt a great deal and grown as a result.

In 1986, while I was studying for Part II of my Obstetric Physiotherapy qualification and researching and writing a paper about 'The role of the obstetric physiotherapist in a Well Woman Centre and a Postnatal Support Group', I first had the idea for a book for women who had become mothers. Later that year when I became a Look After Yourself (LAY) tutor, I realised that a lot of what the LAY package had to offer was particularly relevant to couples embarking on parenthood.

The Look After Yourself project is a government-funded Health Education Authority project, aimed at raising peoples' awareness about the various lifestyle factors which relate to coronary heart disease in an attempt to encourage people to take responsibility for their own health and adopt a healthier lifestyle. LAY offers information about exercise, healthy eating, smoking, sensible alcohol consumption and stress management which includes relaxation skills. It was certainly very beneficial to me personally in learning more about what stress is, and how to deal with it effectively.

In 1989, I was fortunate enough to be asked to attend an international conference in Amsterdam, on Psychosomatic Obstetrics and Gynaecology on behalf of the National Childbirth Trust. Many of the lectures that I heard there gave me food for thought.

The title of the conference was "The Free Woman; Women's Health in the 1990's." The Conference Chairman in his opening address, drew attention to the link between women's emancipation and their health and the fact that to become a free woman you need good health and that you need to be a free woman to obtain good health care. Many of the speakers I heard, confirmed for me the overwhelming need there is for women to have more information to be able to take responsibility for their own health and to enable them to obtain appropriate medical care.

Over the past three years I have been involved in a pilot scheme to train NCT postnatal exercise teachers. This pilot scheme has been successfully completed and there are now a number of postnatal exercise and discussion classes being held all over the country. The number of new teachers will gradually grow so that more and more new mothers will have an opportunity to attend an exercise class planned specifically with them in mind. It has been as a result of my involvement with this pilot scheme that this book has finally become a reality.

It would not have been possible without the considerable help and encouragement I have received from so many different people. My special thanks go to Mary Newburn of the NCT and Fiona MacIntyre of Ebury Press for all their support and encouragement as the book gradually took shape. I have really appreciated the helpful comments made by Sally Crompton, Sue Bruton, Pam Bartlett and

Anne Pegum of the NCT on everything I wrote, as I went along. They really helped me to re-shape areas when I got bogged down with the writing.

Thanks are due to others who so generously shared their specific expertise and knowledge; obstetric physiotherapists Mollie Jennings and Marion Grant; Judy Di Fiore, an exercise teacher and trainer for the Y.M.C.A., on the exercise section; Shirleyanne Seel on the breastfeeding section; Karen Munro, a state registered dietician, on the sensible eating section and Sue Rickells, Jo O'Farrell, Yvonne Rowe, Veronica Lewis and Liz Hargest for their help on the chapter of the book for mothers with a disability.

I would like to thank all those mothers who agreed to be photographed with their lovely babies for the book. I am sure you will agree that they help make all the exercises clear for the reader. My thanks go to all those women who shared their experiences of what being a mother has meant to them and to Sally Crompton and Diz Meredith for collecting the quotes.

During the past year, I have especially enjoyed working on the Ante and Postnatal exercise courses at the YMCA Training and Development Department and have learnt a great deal from the people I have worked with there, especially Jill Gaskell, Susie Dinan and Judy Di Fiore.

My thanks to Paul White and Ann Aris, my LAY colleagues for all their support and the generous way in which they shared their knowledge and experience. I have learnt so much from them both. Last but not least, there are my dear friends Ave Houston and Sandra Silvester who encouraged me to believe that I could do it when I doubted. To my wonderful husband David and three sons, Andrew, Robert and Richard I owe the most. Only they know what it was really like living with me as the deadline drew nearer and nearer. I thank you for all your loving support throughout the whole project.

A number of the women whom I met while preparing to write this book, commented on how much closer to their own mothers they felt once they had become a mother themselves. While writing this book and talking to a number of mothers with a disability, I have thought a lot about my own mother, Pat Gush, and the way she coped with two small children despite being partially paralysed. She died when I was eleven, so we never had an opportunity to be able to share and compare our experiences of motherhood together. This book is written in loving memory of her.

GILLIAN FLETCHER

· · · · ·

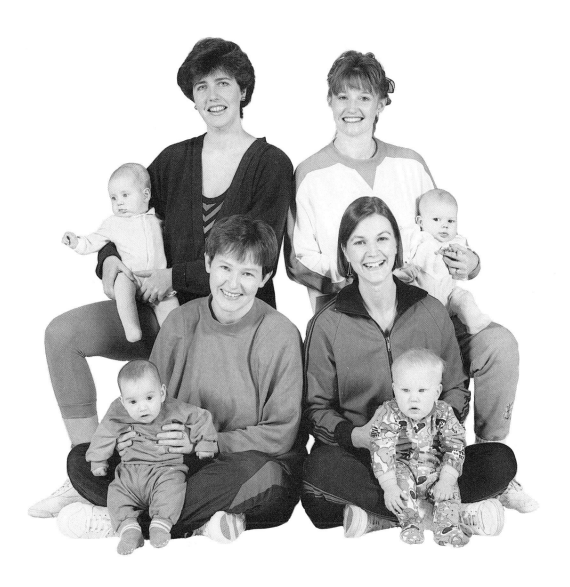

The models in the photographs in this book are, from
top left clockwise, Abbé Lyle and baby Emma,
Linda Tranter and baby Sarah, Gillian Clough Rusling
and baby Stephen and Gerlinde Nanda and baby
Hannah.

Introduction

Becoming a mother, especially for the first time, is a momentous experience and one women never forget. However much you read and discuss, or even experience motherhood at secondhand through close friends or sisters, before the birth of your baby, nothing can really prepare you for the powerful reality of being a mother. The warm feelings can be sheer magic, releasing strong emotions of love and tenderness as if some untapped well within you has been suddenly uncapped.

These personal and individual feelings are very hard to describe to someone who has not experienced motherhood. The traditional image of motherhood – the serene and contented mother with a clean and rosy infant in her arms – is only one side of the story.

While transition to motherhood is smooth and easy for some, others find it a real shock. Many women have an idealised picture of motherhood built up in their minds but unfortunately the physical and emotional difficulties they experience are so far removed from that picture that they are left feeling bewildered, frustrated and often guilty and lacking in confidence because of their 'failure' to cope with something they thought would be the most natural thing in the world.

The down side of mothering can be worse than you had anticipated. You may experience more frustration, tiredness and anxiety than you had imagined possible. Initially it seems as if your whole being is focussed on this small, damp and helpless person you have just met for the first time, even though you may feel you have known her for many months while she grew inside you. You may be overwhelmed by the responsibility of it all and suddenly become aware of your own emotional vulnerability, recognising the very strong feelings that this baby can cause in you.

During pregnancy, you probably spent some time daydreaming about your child and the sort of mothering you might be able to give her. This idea of a 'possible mother' is then tested in the early months against the reality of the 'actual mother' you become or are allowed to become. For many women there seems to be a worryingly large gap between the two, and the tendency then is to try harder to become the sort of mother you thought you could be.

Many mothers fall into the trap of trying to be the perfect mother and devote themselves selflessly to this task, allowing the baby to become their life and often neglecting their own needs and interests. This is largely due to a feeling that the time of babyhood is short, but also guilt borne of the belief that the family should always come first. Having a tireless slave of a mother, always at her beck and call, can be quite a burden for a child as she grows older and starts to develop her own independence. Learning that her mother has rights as an individual, independent of her role as a mother can be a valuable part of growing up.

Being realistic about the situation will help you to get things into perspective and allow yourself to become a 'good enough mother'. It is important to remember that mothering is a two-way interaction between you and your baby, who is a unique individual right from birth. To a greater or lesser extent each child determines the parenting she will receive by her responses. Remember it is not all down to you alone.

It is probably one of the most complex roles you will ever have, very rewarding but equally very demanding and frustrating, and one which is for life – unlike other relationships, which can be ended by divorce, moving house, changing jobs etc. Because of this and the importance which most people attribute to the role, women invest an enormous amount of emotional energy into 'getting it right' AND liking it.

Modern contraceptive measures which enable people to decide whether or not to have children and when to have them, can seem to add to the burden. It is hard to admit to finding life extremely difficult and not as fulfilling or enjoyable as you had hoped, when your situation is the result of a positive choice made by you and your partner. A conspiracy of silence among mothers is also more likely to make a new mother feel as if she is the only one not coping, when everyone else appears to be enjoying motherhood and coping marvellously.

Having a baby changes a woman's life in all kinds of ways. It is a period of enormous adjustment which is both challenging and frightening. We feel secure and that our lives are well ordered when we are surrounded by familiar and safe structure and routine. Change of any kind causes stress and a new mother has to cope with a number of different changes in her life all at once.

There are not only the physical changes of recovering from pregnancy, labour and delivery but also the emotional changes involved in becoming a mother and the changing relationship with her partner now that the couple have become a family. For some it also coincides with a period of adjustment from being a financially independent working woman to being a full time housewife and mother, financially dependent on her partner, losing the day-to-day contact with her work colleagues as well as suffering the loss of status.

Women who intend to return to paid work, often spend a good deal of their time during the early days worrying about organising suitable childcare arrangements, and wondering how they and their babies will cope.

Being a mother has been likened to one of those circus jugglers who sets a number of plates spinning, each one on the end of a tall pole, and then has to keep running up and down the line twirling the poles to keep all the plates from falling to the ground. Anyone who is already a mother will recognise the analogy immediately, knowing that a mother is expected to be comforter and mentor, teacher, nurse and nanny, as well as skilled at sewing, cooking, shopping, cleaning, gardening and managing the household. A job description could also include the requirement to do several of these activities at the same time and that she probably has to meet the needs of a partner as well. The working hours could be flexible providing she is prepared to be on duty for any of the 24 hours in a day. No salary is offered for this job as the satisfaction of the job is thought to be reward enough.

If a mother has a disability, she has the added difficulty of coping with lack of information, specific to her needs, as well as dealing with feelings of isolation in not being able to meet other mothers in a similar

> **❝❝I don't think anyone anywhere could have prepared me for some of the postnatal feelings. At times I felt almost overwhelmed by this little thing who didn't fall neatly into any of my 'filing trays' and allow me to implement my time management training. At times I found it hard to accept that I 'the professional woman, manager of people' could be so weak, so ineffectual.❞❞**

situation very easily. Adjusting to motherhood without suitably adapted equipment, or the help of health professionals who understand the limitations of her disability, can make life very difficult for the new mother with a disability.

The early weeks of motherhood are probably the most stressful. Understanding a little more about the nature of stress and how it affects you, will help you to learn to cope with it more easily.

Stress means different things to different people. Most people think of it as a negative force. Some think of it as circumstances or situations which cause them problems and over which they have little or no control. Others describe it as the feelings of tension, anxiety, being rushed and overworked which they experience in certain situations. In reality, it can be positive, as we all need a certain amount of stimulation and challenge to enable us to function effectively.

It is when we feel there is an imbalance between the DEMANDS placed upon us in any situation and our ABILITY to cope with those demands that stress becomes harmful and out of control. The key factor here is our own 'perception'. This may explain why some people thrive in certain situations which others might see as particularly stressful. For example a deadline inspires and challenges some to greater productivity while it may cause panic and inability to function in another person.

Seeing stress as simply an imbalance between demands and capability can be very helpful because it changes you from a passive victim of your circumstances to someone who has some control. You may not be able to alter the demands placed upon you but you can learn to recognise and register them, analyse them and your responses to them and if necessary alter your response to them. You can also learn to lessen the other demands placed upon you at a time when you are having to deal with a major crisis or demand in your life. You do not have to be on call all the time doing everything just because that is what you have always done. It is possible to change the way you behave.

In this book the chapter on your changing role, suggests ways of recognising the stresses in your life, realising what your response usually is and possible alternative responses that you could try. Goal setting and time planning suggestions are also included as well as some basic relaxation techniques.

Many women are also called upon to care for elderly relatives. If this happens when their children are small it can be especially difficult. With current government policies encouraging care in the community, this trend will increase. All these demands upon a woman often lead to her neglecting her own health in favour of providing unstinting care for her family.

Good health is more than just not being ill, it is a very positive attribute which most people take for granted until they lose it. The World Health Organisation defines it as "a state of complete mental, physical and social well-being and not merely the absence of disease." Women tend to suffer ill health to a greater extent than men for reasons that are not always clear. Some illness is of a gynaecological nature, specific to women, but they also seem to suffer more from certain diseases which also affect men.

Many of the problems women encounter in

> **❝Since the birth of my baby, the professionals have, quite rightly so, been more concerned about his welfare and I have tended not to bother them with my own physical and emotional problems.❞**

trying to obtain good health care stem from the fact that many of the health care providers and most of the policy makers are men, who cannot identify directly with women's health problems and needs.

The natural experiences of women's lives such as menstruation, pregnancy, childbirth and the menopause have all been 'medicalised', leading women to believe that they require the full panoply of the medical profession to help them through these stages of life, as if through an illness. Women have been encouraged for too long to look to others for the solutions to their problems when much of the solution lies with the woman herself if only she will recognise it and take responsibility for managing her lifestyle in such a way as to maximise her health and minimise any potential problems.

This book aims to give women the information they need to lead a healthier lifestyle and take effective charge of some of the areas of their lives which cause them stress. It includes postnatal exercise for the first few days after the birth, as well as a range of stronger exercises to include as you get fitter. There is advice on coping with stress and adjusting to your new role as a mother with additional information for mothers with a disability. General information on sensible eating and weight control, returning to work and keeping healthy is also included, and throughout the book there are quotes from many women who so kindly agreed to share their experiences as mothers. In this book the baby is referred to as she while the older child or toddler is referred to as he.

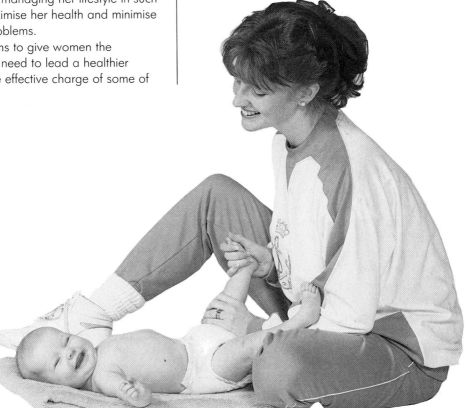

The first few weeks

The early days following the birth of your baby are full of surprises and a mixture of many emotions. There is the tiredness and relief that it is all over and the baby has safely arrived; the excitement and joy of getting to know her plus all the uncertainties and anxieties about your new role and the demands that will be placed upon you.

While the new baby inevitably becomes the focus of attention, it is important to remember that you also have needs. It takes times to adjust to the many changes brought about by the birth of your baby. Take the time to enjoy the baby and don't expect too much of yourself too soon.

You will probably be keen to regain your former pre-pregnancy shape and size so that you can get back into clothes you haven't worn for months. This chapter contains a whole programme of exercises to help you get back in shape, and the sooner you start exercising the sooner you will recover from the birth and begin the return to normal. The most important exercises are starred – these are the ones you should start on as soon as possible.

The childbearing years are the years during which many women develop an awareness of their body that they may never have had before, and after a few months of postnatal exercising they may well find themselves fitter than before they became pregnant.

During pregnancy your body goes through some remarkable changes as it adjusts to the increasing weight and size of the baby and prepares for the birth, but these changes happen gradually over the months and so you have time to get used to them.

However, in the early days following the birth your body goes through a number of quite dramatic and rapid physical changes as it returns to normal and at the same time starts to produce breastmilk for your baby, a process which begins in pregnancy and is triggered into action by the birth. All of this can make you feel strangely out of touch with your body at times. Understanding why these changes are occurring may make them easier to cope with.

THE ABDOMINAL MUSCLES

You may be surprised at just how stretched and flabby your abdomen seems in the early days following the birth, but it isn't so surprising when you think that during pregnancy your waist measurement may have increased by as much as 50 cm (20 inches), and it is going to take a little time and effort for these muscles to recover and regain their former shape and strength.

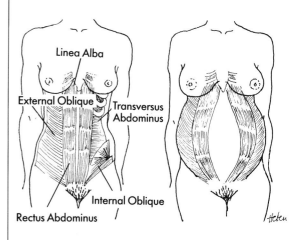

Linea Alba

External Oblique

Transversus Abdominus

Internal Oblique

Rectus Abdominus

BEFORE PREGNANCY

DURING PREGNANCY

The abdominal muscles (nature's corset) consist of four interlacing muscle layers which perform a number of important functions:
• They protect the abdominal contents including the pregnant uterus.
• They support the spine and maintain the correct pelvic tilt.
• They move the trunk in different directions.
• They aid the body in expulsive activities such as in childbirth, coughing and sneezing.

On the surface and running straight up and down the middle are the rectus abdominus muscles which consist of the two halves joined by a thin fibrous band called the linea alba. At the sides are two layers which run obliquely across the abdomen in different directions and a deep layer which runs from side to side across the front. Some of these layers do not come all the way across to the centre. Down the middle the abdomen is only one muscle layer thick which makes it weaker and more vulnerable.

During pregnancy, softening and stretching of the linea alba occurs, allowing the rectus abdominus muscle bands to separate to accommodate the growing baby. This separation is known as diastasis rectii.

Immediately after the birth for about 3–4 days you may be able to feel a space of two–four finger widths. As the muscle strength improves this gap begins to close and should eventually narrow until it is so small that it is only about the width of the tip of one of your fingers.

You can help this process by doing some simple specific exercises as soon as possible, progressing to more strenuous exercises as the muscles regain their shape and strength. Before doing some of the exercises in this book, you need to do the simple check below to see how well your muscles are returning to normal (the individual exercises state where this is necessary).

The Rec Check ☆

To do this check accurately you need to make the muscles work strongly.

Lie on your back with your knees bent and your feet flat on the bed or floor. Pull in your abdominal muscles and lift your head and shoulders off the bed while stretching one hand towards your feet. Place the fingers of your other hand just below your umbilicus (tummy button) and feel for the two firm ridges of the rectus muscles which should be working hard.

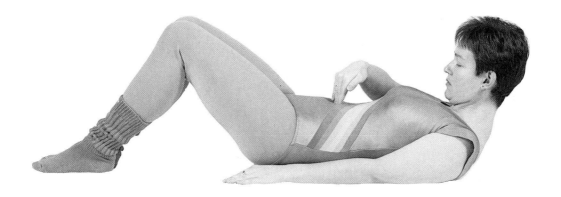

THE UTERUS

The uterus is a bag of criss-crossing muscle fibres and during pregnancy, under the influence of the hormones released by your body, it gradually stretches to accommodate the growing baby. These changes are quite remarkable when you think that the uterus enlarges from its pre-pregnant size of a small pear to the size of a large water melon, and its weight increases from about 60 grams (2 ounces) to about 1000 grams (2½ lb)!

Following the birth of the baby and the expulsion of the placenta, the uterus is considerably smaller but it takes about six weeks for it to shrink back to its original size and weight. This shrinking process is called involution. During involution, the lining of the uterus, which is no longer needed, is shed. The discharge, called lochia, lasts for three–four weeks. It is initially red blood coming mainly from the placental site. After a few days it becomes brown in colour and after a few weeks turns yellowish white. The colour change is unpredictable due to great variations in the amount of blood loss over this period. Small blood clots are quite common. Normal lochia does not smell offensive. If you notice large blood clots, a persistent or excessive loss, or one which has an offensive smell, you should tell your midwife or doctor. It may mean that you have an infection in your uterus and treatment will be required.

After-pains

'After-pains' are caused by the contractions of the uterus as it shrinks back to normal. The contractions are brought on by the release of the hormone oxytocin, which is also responsible for letting down the milk in the breasts. Oxytocin is automatically produced when you put the baby to the breast, so you may be more aware of these pains and increased loss of lochia when you breastfeed. Strong after-pains are more common in women having second or subsequent babies than those having their first baby. It is important to recognise that they are part of a normal process. You will have less discomfort if you relax and breathe through them rather than tense up. After-pains usually only last for a few days.

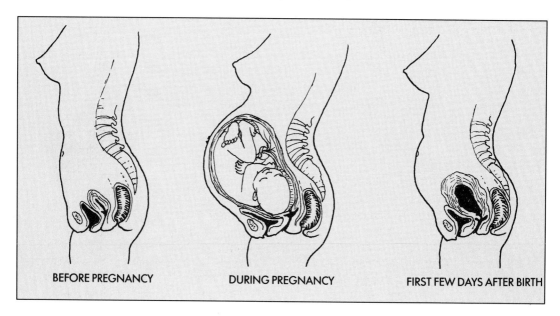

BEFORE PREGNANCY   DURING PREGNANCY   FIRST FEW DAYS AFTER BIRTH

PELVIC FLOOR MUSCLES

The pelvis is a bony basin which consists of two big pelvic bones which join the base of the spine (the sacrum) at the back at two joints called the sacroiliac joints. The pelvic bones connect together at the front at a joint called the pubic symphysis. At the very base of the spine below the sacrum are four small bones fused together to form the coccyx or tail bone.

The pelvis provides the main support structure for the body and protects the uterus and bladder and, in early pregnancy, the growing foetus. Forming the floor of this basin is a hammock of muscles called the pelvic floor. It is divided into two layers, one deep and one superficial, attached from the pubic symphysis at the front to the coccyx at the back and across to the hip bones at the sides.

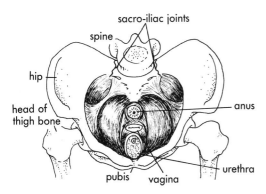

The pelvic floor

Women have three openings in these muscles, one at the front from the bladder (the urethral opening), one in the middle from the uterus (the vaginal opening) and one, at the back, from the large bowel (the anal opening).

There are loops of extra muscle around these openings called sphincters which normally contract to keep the openings tightly closed, especially when the pressure in the abdomen is raised, such as when you cough, laugh or sneeze. During pregnancy, the pelvic muscles support all the extra weight of the baby, the placenta and all the fluid inside the enlarged uterus. During the birth these muscles will have been considerably stretched and weakened, so you will need to exercise them as soon, and as often, as possible to encourage them to become strong again.

If you have had stitches from a tear or an episiotomy (a cut which is sometimes made to enlarge the vaginal opening during birth) you may be afraid to tighten the muscles because of pain. When you tighten and relax the muscles you improve the blood supply and this will help with the healing process. You can't do any harm to the stitches by exercising, so the sooner you start the better.

You will already be familiar with how to exercise your pelvic floor without perhaps realising it. Every time you feel the need to empty your bladder and it is not convenient to do so you contract your pelvic floor muscles to prevent you passing urine.

THE BLADDER

You will find that you need to empty your bladder frequently in the early days after the birth, as the body gets rid of extra fluid. Some women have difficulty in passing urine after childbirth. This may be due to stretching and bruising of the urethra (the passage leading from the bladder to the exterior) and occasionally a catheter may be needed until the bladder has returned to normal. If you have had an epidural during labour, you may need a catheter in position for a few hours after the birth.

A more common problem following childbirth is stress incontinence. This is an involuntary loss of urine that occurs when the pressure inside the abdomen is increased when coughing, laughing or sneezing. Pelvic floor exercises, started as soon as possible and continued as often as possible, are an important factor in correcting this distressing condition, and women who do other exercises regularly as well as doing their pelvic floor contractions have fewer problems than those who just do a few pelvic floor contractions or no exercise at all.

If, after doing your pelvic floor exercises correctly and frequently for several weeks, you show no signs of improvement in your bladder control, ask your GP to refer you to an obstetric physiotherapist for further treatment. Some women may need an operation to repair a 'prolapse' – a condition in which a weakened vaginal wall allows either the uterus, bladder or rectum to sag into an unnatural position.

There are other types of urinary incontinence that cannot be helped by pelvic floor exercises and it is important that these are accurately diagnosed and treated. Do seek help if you think you need it. Don't feel that just because you have had a baby you have to put up with this or any other distressing condition. Help is available, it is just a question of finding the correct treatment for your situation.

THE PERINEUM

The perineum is the area of skin and muscle which lies between the vagina and the anus. If you have had stitches or have a lot of bruising due to pressure from the baby's head during delivery, your perineum may be quite painful in the first few days. Here are some ideas which might help.

Spend some time during the day resting on your tummy as this helps alleviate the pressure for a while. Place a pillow under your head and neck and another under your tummy with a gap for your breasts. Be careful not to squash your breasts in case the pressure causes a blocked duct.

Lie on your side in bed or sit on a rubber ring to feed the baby as this will remove some of the pressure, but don't sit on a ring for long periods of time as it can lead to more swelling in the perineum.

Many people find arnica tablets, which are a homeopathic remedy for bruising and trauma, are helpful.

Sitting well forward on the lavatory or squatting when you pass urine helps prevent excessive stinging.

Have a look at your stitches with a small mirror. You will probably find that they are not nearly as bad as you had imagined.

Basic pelvic floor contractions as described on page 27, started as soon as possible, will help to speed recovery.

Keeping the perineal area clean and dry is important for reducing the risk of infection. Do make sure that the bath, lavatory and bidet are thoroughly cleaned before you use them, especially while still in hospital, as the chances of infection are higher than in your own home. You could take a supply of alcohol toilet wipes or disposable toilet seat covers into hospital with you to be absolutely sure.

> **❛❛I had a forceps delivery and a massive episiotomy. I couldn't sit comfortably for weeks (6-8), I had pain and discomfort for months and became quite depressed about it. I felt very alone with this problem for a good few weeks until I met some other people who were still having perineal problems sometime after the birth. If you have a vaginal delivery, stitches are rarely discussed and still more rarely taken seriously.**

If you use a bidet or hand held shower to clean the perineum, do make sure that the water jets spray from front to back otherwise you can wash faecal material from the anus onto the perineum. You should also make sure you wipe from front to back, to avoid touching the vaginal area with toilet paper that has been in contact with the anus.

In hospital, sanitary towels should be kept in a closed plastic bag inside your locker and carefully disposed of. For further information about avoiding infection see the NCT booklet *Postnatal Infection*.

Haemorrhoids

These are varicose veins around the anus which are caused by:
• The hormonal changes of pregnancy, which allow the vein walls to become stretched.
• The increased pressure inside the pelvis during pregnancy and delivery.

Some women experience problems with varicose veins around the vaginal opening. These are known as vulval varicose veins.

Pelvic floor exercises will help by increasing the circulation to the area which will speed up the healing. You may also find some relief from the application of a cream to help relieve the swelling and pain, so do tell someone if they are causing you problems.

Constipation and straining to open your bowels should be avoided as this puts further strain on the varicose veins. If you have stitches, holding a folded pad of toilet paper over them when you open your bowels will be more comfortable. Make sure you get enough fibre in your diet and drink plenty of fluids.

• • • • • •

CAESAREAN SECTION

If you have had a Caesarean section you may find that in the first few days you are preoccupied with the discomfort of the incision and the difficulties of moving around, finding a comfortable position for feeding the baby and getting in and out of bed. For many women the fear of the pain or the stitches not holding makes matters worse. Tension caused by fear will only increase your pain. You may feel inclined to stoop forwards to try to protect your incision but you should stand as straight as possible while walking around, relax and breathe comfortably, supporting the area gently with one hand.

Finding a comfortable position in which to feed your baby may be a matter of trial and error. Supporting the baby with a pillow on your lap may protect your scar and you may find that sitting in a chair is easier than on the bed (see the NCT leaflet *Breastfeeding after a Caesarean section*).

You will need help getting in and out of bed initially, and it is important that anyone helping you out of bed lets you move at your own pace and doesn't try to pull you up into a sitting position suddenly. Support your incision with one hand and bend your knees, then roll over on to your side keeping both knees together and your shoulders and hips in a straight line to avoid twisting. Push yourself up into a sitting position and as you do so let your legs swing slowly down over the side of the bed and onto the floor. Hopefully your bed will be about the right height for your feet to touch the floor and you can then push yourself up into a standing position. If not, slowly lower yourself off the side of the bed until your feet reach the floor, or ask for the height of the bed to be adjusted.

> **❝I hadn't expected piles — the pain just makes you weep. It's not a very nice subject.❞**

To get back into bed, sit yourself as near to the head of the bed as possible and, bracing your abdominal muscles, ease your legs one at a time onto the bed. You may need to lift your legs with your hands. Keeping your knees bent, dig your heels into the bed and push yourself back towards the head of the bed with your hands.

All the exercises for the first six weeks (see page 24) are perfectly safe for you to perform if you have had a Caesarean section but you should wait 10–12 weeks before starting on the major exercise programme in this book. On page 31, there are some additional exercises you should include in the first few days after a Caesarean section to improve your circulation as you are likely to be less mobile, and if you have a general anaesthetic you should do some deep breathing and coughing to help clear away any secretions in your lungs. Secretions are produced as a reaction to the anaesthetic and, because it is painful to cough with an abdominal incision, you tend to suppress your body's normal instinct to get rid of them. Left in the lungs they may cause infection.

A blind mother with five children, all of whom were breastfed:

66 Apart from initial difficulties with latching on, I had no real problems. It was always more convenient as I couldn't see to mix bottles of formula. I really enjoy the closeness with the baby and being able to meet his needs and knowing that I've given him the best possible start. 99

BREASTS

As soon as your baby is born, hormones stimulate the breasts to start the milk production process. For the first few days breasts continue to produce colostrum as they did in pregnancy. Colostrum has a higher protein content than mature breast milk and is important in sustaining the baby until the milk comes in. It is rich in antibodies which help protect against infection and allergy.

Most mothers find breastfeeding a pleasurable experience, but in the early days there may be a number of minor difficulties which may make you feel very unsure about the whole experience. It takes time to learn this new skill and it is worth knowing how to minimise potential problems. Your nipples may be very sensitive at first and it is important to prevent them becoming really sore.

Position the baby at the breast so that she is on her side with her chest and tummy towards you. Ensure that she is not just sucking on the end of the nipple but has a good deal of the areola in her mouth. To be able to do that she needs to be able to tilt her head back and touch the breast with her chin so that she can open her mouth properly. Don't hold her too close to the breast. When she is on properly you will see the muscles at her temples and her ears wiggling as she sucks. If your baby is correctly positioned you shouldn't get sore, although some mothers experience discomfort for the first few days.

Support your breast from underneath with a hand flat against your ribcage. Avoid pressing the top of your breast with your finger as this points the nipple in the wrong direction and can cause a blocked duct.

Let your baby decide on the length of feeds and the interval between them.

If your baby is feeding well there should be no need to take her off the breast, but if you want to change her position, gently release her from the breast by placing the tip of your little finger in the corner of her mouth to break the suction which can be surprisingly strong.

Alternate the breasts so that at each feed you start on a different side. Don't worry if your baby only feeds from one breast and then falls asleep. In the early days, many babies have only one breast at each feed. Changing your baby's position at different feeds also helps avoid one area of the breast getting too much pressure.

If your nipples feel tender, rubbing some expressed breast milk into them at the end of the feed can help keep them supple.

About 3–5 days after the birth the milk comes in. (It may take longer if you have had a general anaesthetic). You may find that your breasts are suddenly very hot, swollen and hard. This condition, known as primary engorgement, is due to an increased blood supply and the milk which is now being produced. It can be uncomfortable but is only temporary and will soon pass.

The following are all ideas which may help:
• Encourage the baby to feed for as long as she wants before changing sides and feed her when she asks.
• Before a feed, splash warm water over the breasts to help get the milk flowing, so that the baby is not struggling to feed from a hard, painful breast.
• If the breast is hard, gently hand express some milk so the baby can feed more easily.
• Applying ice cold flannels to your breasts immediately after a feed will constrict the blood vessels and help reduce some of the swelling, as well as cooling them.
• Gently stroking some of the swelling away from the nipple will help as well.
• A good firm supporting bra will make your breasts feel more comfortable. Mava bras are available from NCT Maternity Sales (see Useful Addresses, page 139).

For further information on breastfeeding the following NCT leaflets are available from NCT

Maternity Sales: *Breastfeeding – a good start, Breastfeeding – avoiding some of the problems, Breastfeeding after a Caesarean section, How to express and store breast milk, Breastfeeding if your baby needs special care.*

POSTURE

The changes which occurred in your body during pregnancy altered your centre of gravity, weakened certain muscles, increased your weight and softened your ligaments. Immediately after the birth of your baby, all these changes start to be reversed and you have to learn to adjust to a new you. It may take a little while to re-orientate your posture to a non-pregnant state as you have probably got so used to carrying a baby, and with weak abdominal muscles your pelvis may be tipped forward causing backache either in the lower back or between the shoulder blades.

Posture is mainly controlled by reflexes but it can also be influenced by factors such as fatigue, muscle weakness and mood. It is important to be aware of your posture and any faults that you may have developed during the pregnancy, so that you can make the necessary adjustments. If you don't, you may find yourself dogged by constant muscle fatigue and tension and, in the long term, this can lead to more wear and tear on your joints.

Think of standing as tall as you can with the weight evenly distributed on both feet. Keep your knees soft and not locked straight. Pull in your abdominal muscles and tuck your bottom in and under, so that you correct the tilt of your pelvis. Press your shoulders down and back and lengthen the back of your neck by tucking your chin in. Good posture means balancing one part of the body with another and minimising the amount of muscular effort required to maintain that position.

HOW TO AVOID BACKACHE

Backache is one of the most common problems encountered during pregnancy and in the early months after the birth. During pregnancy, large amounts of the hormone relaxin are present in the body. This makes the ligaments soften and become more elastic and pliable, primarily to enable the joints of the pelvis to widen and separate ready for the birth of the baby. It takes 3–5 months after the birth for the relaxin levels to go back to normal. During this period it is important that you take great care to protect your back from injury. The weakened abdominal muscles are not able to carry out their normal role of protecting the spine, and the increased elasticity in the ligaments of the back and the pelvis makes you particularly vulnerable to back strain when bending, lifting and carrying.

Sitting

Sit well back in your chair, possibly with a small cushion in the small of the back to maintain a good position for the lower back. When your baby is very little, place her on a pillow on your lap. This prevents you from getting too tense in the shoulder region.

Standing

When standing for any length of time you may find that your lower back aches. Lifting one foot slightly higher than the other allows you to release some tension in the lower back. If your sink is too low and causes your back to ache, try using a washing up bowl resting on another one turned upside down in the sink.

Lifting

If you have a toddler it may be helpful to lift him to your own level before doing things like tying up shoelaces, or kneel down to his level rather than stooping. If you are going to pick him up, bend your knees with one foot placed in front of the other, brace your pelvic floor and abdominal muscles and breathe out as you lift. Kneel down to bath him and encourage him to do as much as he can to help you.

Carrying

It is much better to carry your baby in a sling in front of you than perched on one hip which puts more strain on your back.

When shopping, try to carry your goods in two evenly weighted bags, one in each hand, rather than one large bag. Use a back pack if you are pushing the pram and have too much shopping for the pram tray.

Choose a pram or buggy the right height for you. Your hands resting on the handles should be level with your iliac crests about 5–7 cm (2–3 inches) below your waist.

Changing Nappies

The work surface you use for changing your baby's nappies will be used many, many times before the baby is old enough not to need them, and it is important that it is the right height. Try to choose a surface the same height as the buggy handles, and remember to keep a close watch on the baby because they are able to roll over much sooner than you think.

HOW TO MANAGE BACKACHE

If in spite of all your precautions you do get backache, you need to do all you can to alleviate any symptoms as soon as possible. Also try to identify what in particular caused it so that you can avoid it happening again.

Mild discomfort may be due to poor posture and tension or generalised fatigue. Check your posture and make sure you are following the guidelines for protecting your back. Try to purposefully relax into whatever position you happen to be working in, concentrating on letting go any unnecessary tension. THE EMPHASIS SHOULD ALWAYS BE ON ECONOMY OF EFFORT.

In a recent survey in the British Medical Journal, (see References on page 142), it was reported that about 8% of women who had used an epidural as a means of pain relief during labour, suffered from long-term postnatal backache which could be directly attributed to the epidural. Women having epidural Caesarean sections were not affected in this way.

It seems the possible cause was straining of ligaments and nerve pressure in the back during labour. Pain is usually a danger signal which makes us stop doing something which is likely to cause us damage. With an epidural, the total absence of pain allows a situation to continue, which can result in the straining of muscles.

It is important that mothers, partners and staff present at delivery are all aware of the potential danger and that they try to ensure that the labouring woman is in a good postural position on the delivery bed.

If you have pain in your lower back (at the sacro-iliac joints) a soak in a hot bath whatever the time of day can be wonderfully relaxing and refreshing and can ease away the pain in no time instead of allowing it to get progressively worse throughout the day. If it's what you need, try not to feel guilty about taking time out for yourself. You can do this while your baby is asleep or she will probably lie happily on a towel on the floor beside you. If you have a toddler, he will think it's a wonderful opportunity for some water play in the basin with a few beakers, or you could have the toddler or baby in the bath with you.

Lying down may help alleviate the pain or discomfort, but if you find that you wake up with a stiff back, it may be your bed that's at fault. Some beds are far too soft to provide adequate support for your back. Buying a new bed is very costly but a simple remedy is to place a piece of hardboard across the frame under the mattress. If you sleep on your side and the back pain seems to be mainly in the area of your sacro-iliac joint, try placing a cushion or a rolled towel under the top leg when you sleep.

Any back pain which is severe or persistent should be investigated by your GP as back problems can become chronic long-term problems which are very difficult to correct.

Try some of the back pain exercises on pages 28 and 29 to get rid of the waste products caused by unnecessary muscle tension. These exercises should be performed slowly and rhythmically and shouldn't cause any pain.

> **66** *When she sleeps in the morning I get on and prepare the evening meal and any other little chores that are easier when she is not around. When she sleeps in the afternoon I rest.* **99**

• • • • •

GETTING DOWN ONTO THE FLOOR

Whenever you get down onto and up from the floor to exercise it is important to take care to avoid any unnecessary twisting movements.

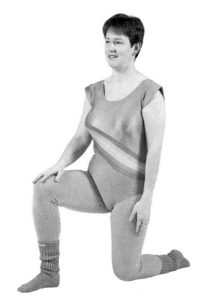

1 Lower yourself down onto one knee.

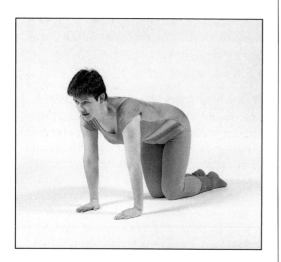

2 Then lower yourself onto both knees.

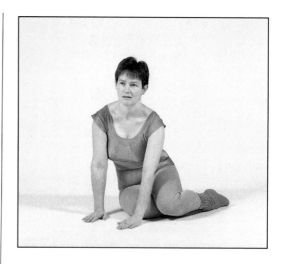

3 With your hands on the floor in front of you, carefully lower yourself down into a side sitting position.

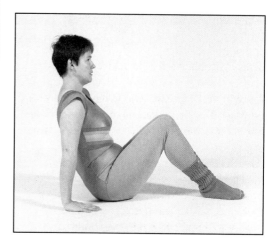

4 Swing your legs round in front of you and lower yourself down into a lying position while keeping your knees bent.

    To get up, roll from your back onto your side with knees bent. Push yourself up into a side sitting position and then into an all-fours kneeling position. Place one foot in front of you on the ground in a half-kneeling position with your hands resting on the bent thigh. Push yourself up into a standing position.

ADOMINAL MUSCLE EXERCISES

Pelvic Rocking ☆

This is a very useful exercise which you may be familiar with from your antenatal classes. It improves posture and is helpful if you suffer from post-Caesarean section pain.

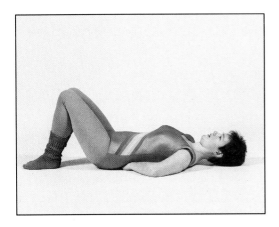

Lie on your back with your knees together and bent, feet flat on the bed or floor. Place one hand under the small of your back and feel the slight gap. Breathe in and then, as you breath out, pull in your abdominal muscles, and press the small of your back flat towards the bed against your hand. Hold for a count of 4 and then release. Repeat frequently and as the muscle strength improves you can hold for longer. Once you have the feel of this movement it can be done sitting or standing to ease backache. You can then also do a pelvic floor contraction (see page 27) with this abdominal one.

• • • • • •

Leg Sliding ☆

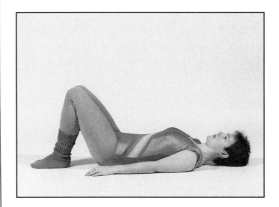

1 Lie on your back with your knees together and bent, feet flat on the bed. Breathe in and as you breathe out, pull your abdominal muscles in as for the pelvic rocking exercise.

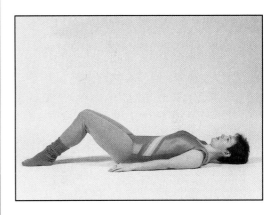

2 Hold the muscles firmly contracted and keep your feet flat on the bed or floor. Slide your legs away from you, trying to keep your back flat. As soon as your back starts to arch off the bed, slide your legs back up again, bending your knees and pressing the small of the back flat all the time. Repeat the exercise from the beginning again. At first you may find that you are not able to slide your legs very far before your back starts to arch because your muscles are so weak, but as you get stronger you will be able to go further.

Curl-ups ☆

This exercise will help strengthen the rectus abdominus muscles.

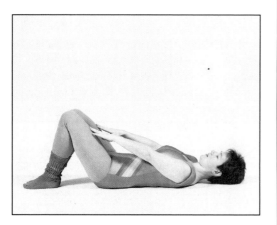

1 Lie on your back with your knees bent and your feet flat on the bed. For the first few weeks it may be advisable to have a pillow under your head.

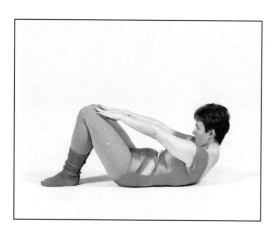

2 Breathe in and as you breathe out, pull in your abdominal muscles, tuck your chin in, and lift your head and shoulders as high as you can off the bed or floor, without allowing your abdomen to bulge or dome. Hold for a count of 4 and then lower. Do 6 or 8 and gradually build up to 10 or 12, sliding the

hands up the thighs as you get stronger. If you feel a strain in your neck, use one hand to support beside your ear. **Do not use both hands** as this makes it a much stronger exercise for the abdominal muscles.

Curl-ups with Wide Separation of Rectus Abdominus Muscles

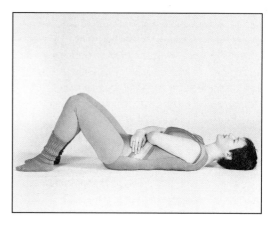

1 If you have a wide separation of the rectus abdominus muscles (see page 15), you should cross both hands over your abdomen (left hand on the right and right hand on the left side, at waist level).

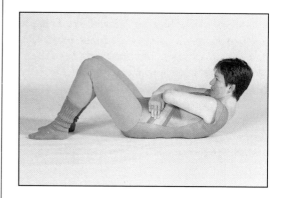

2 As you lift your head up, draw the edges of the muscles together by pulling your hands closer towards each other.

PELVIC FLOOR EXERCISES

The Pelvic Floor Squeeze ☆

In a sitting or lying position, pull up around the back passage and then pull up towards the front passage as if to stop yourself passing urine. Hold the contraction for a count of 4, breathing normally all the time. Release and then repeat another 6 times.

Doing this exercise after each visit to the lavatory will ensure quite a few contractions each day, but you should try to include this important exercise as often as you can especially in the early days (try to do at least 50 a day). Once in a while, check how the muscle strength is improving by trying to stop midstream when passing urine. It is best not to use stopping midstream as a way of doing your pelvic floor exercises on a regular basis, just as an occasional check.

The Lift ☆

Imagine that your pelvic floor is like a lift in a building. Tighten the muscles around the back and front passages as if closing the lift doors tightly. Now tighten a little more as if to take the lift to the second floor. Tighten more as if to reach the third floor and continue until you reach as far as you can go and then gradually descend again to the ground floor. Make sure you don't hold your breath at the same time. By pushing the pelvic floor muscles as if taking the lift down into the basement you may become even more aware of your pelvic floor muscles and what they are capable of, but always make sure you finish with a pull up to the ground floor.

Sexercise ☆

You can enlist your partner's help by gripping his penis with your vaginal muscles as firmly as you can during lovemaking. Don't tell him what you are doing, but when you have contracted the muscles say "Can you feel **that**." If he says "feel **what**?" then you will know that you have quite a lot of work to do in improving the tone of those muscles. With exercise they will improve and he will then be able to give you positive feedback about how they are getting stronger.

Handy Hints

- Always remember **not to hold your breath** when tightening your pelvic floor.
- Concentrate on the quality of the contraction rather than the number. Think about drawing in every muscle fibre each time you contract the muscles.
- Place some coloured dot stickers around the house in strategic places, such as on the bathroom mirror or the telephone, to act as reminders. Each time you catch sight of a coloured sticker, do 5 or 6 pelvic floor contractions. No one will know your secret unless they have also read this book!
- The supermarket checkout, red traffic signals or boring TV programmes all provide good opportunities to fit in a few extra pelvic floor exercises.
- If possible, try to brace the muscles before lifting, coughing, sneezing or laughing.
- Pelvic floor exercises are best done in frequent batches of about 6 contractions at a time.

BACK PAIN EXERCISES

Pelvic Rocking on All-fours ☆

Pelvic rocking, as shown on page 25 can be helpful in alleviating low backache. However, an alternative position is on all-fours as shown here. Your baby can watch while you do this.

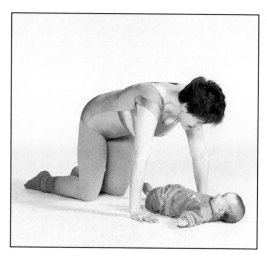

Kneel on the floor with your hands directly under your shoulders and your knees directly under your hips, keeping your back flat. Pull in your abdominal muscles and arch your back towards the ceiling like an angry cat. Keep your head in line with your back. Release and return to the centre, trying to avoid letting your back sag beyond the flat.

You can increase the movement in the lower back and strengthen the back muscles if you pull one knee up towards your nose as you round the back and drop your head and then straighten that leg out behind you. Keep it level with your back, no higher. Bend the knee and replace it on the floor, returning your head to the central position. Repeat 6–8 times and then repeat with the opposite leg another 6–8 times.

• • • • • •

Gentle Leg Rocking

A common site of backache after birth is at the sacro-iliac joints, where the spine joins the pelvis (see page 17). Pain is normally felt just under one of the dimples either side of the spine. The pain may radiate into the whole buttock and there may also be pain down the leg. This exercise is particularly good for relieving this pain in the left sacro-iliac joint; reverse the exercise for the right joint.

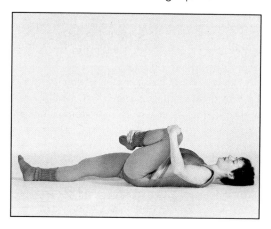

Lie flat on your back with both legs straight and bend the left knee. Keeping your shoulders, head and right leg flat on the floor during the exercise, bend your left knee onto your chest, grasp your left knee with your left hand and place your right hand around your left ankle. Gently pull the knee towards your shoulder with the left hand while pressing the left ankle down towards your pubic bone with your right hand. Slowly release the pressure and repeat the movement a number of times with a gentle rocking motion. Once you have done this exercise it is important that you avoid any twisting movement as you get up.

Replace the left foot flat on the floor with the knee bent. Slowly bend the right knee and place your right foot beside the left one. Keep your knees firmly together and roll onto your side, then push yourself up onto all-fours. Kneel upright on both knees, then half kneel with one foot flat on the floor and carefully get up into a standing position.

If you have low back pain on both sides, lie on your back and bend both knees up onto your chest and hug your knees to your chest, by holding onto your thighs just above the knees. Gently rock from side to side. Follow the instructions above for getting up from the floor carefully.

Arm Circling Backwards ☆

This exercise will help alleviate tension in the large upper back and shoulder girdle muscles and also improve posture.

Stand with your feet about 30 cm (12 inches) apart, keep the knees soft, and not locked back. Make sure your bottom is tucked under and your tummy pulled in. Circle your arms forward and upwards past your ears.

Alternatively, sit on a stool with no back to it and place your feet flat on the floor. Place your hands on your shoulders and circle your elbows up and forwards, round and back, in as large a circle as you comfortably can, brushing close to your ears. Keep the rest of the body still and don't arch your back to compensate for stiff shoulders.

Breathe rhythmically throughout the exercise. Check that your shoulders are down away from your ears after each circle. Repeat 8 –10 times. (Don't circle the arms in a forward direction as this increases the tendency towards round shoulders and poor posture.)

Side Bends ☆

This exercise will make it easier to bend your back from side to side.

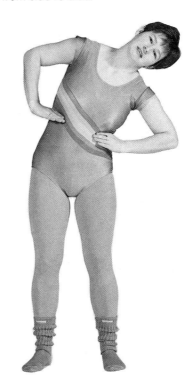

Stand with your feet hip-width apart, and hands on hips, and knees soft. Tighten your abdominal muscles and keep your bottom tucked in. Keeping your hips centred and the weight evenly distributed on both feet, bend smoothly to your left side as far as you comfortably can, hold the position for a few seconds and then repeat to the right side, keeping the body in a straight line as if it were between two panes of glass. Avoid bouncing in an attempt to increase the range of movement as this is counter productive. Alternatively, try sitting with arms down by your side. Breathe out as you bend and in as you recover to a central position. Repeat 8–10 times to each side.

Head, Trunk and Arm Rotating ☆

The movement in the upper spine is mainly one of rotation and is often very limited. This exercise will improve mobility in the upper trunk and shoulder girdle.

Stand tall, with your feet hip-width apart and knees soft, hands and arms stretched out in front of you at shoulder height and shoulder width apart. Tighten your abdominal muscles and keep your bottom tucked in. Keeping your

hips facing the front and your eyes on your left fingertips, turn your head, shoulders and arms around to the left as far as you can go, letting your right arm bend across the chest as you do so. Hold for a few seconds, return to the centre and repeat on the other side. Breathe out as you swing round to one side and in as you return to the centre. Repeat 8–10 times.

Trunk, Knee and Hip Bends

This will make it easier to bend your back backwards and forwards and also make the hip joint more mobile.

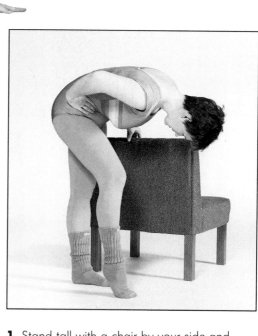

1 Stand tall with a chair by your side and hold onto the back of it with one hand. Keep your knees soft. Raise the heel of your right foot slightly off the floor and curl your head and trunk down towards your right knee. Breathe out as you go down. Hold the position for a few seconds and slowly uncurl to an upright position breathing in as you do so.

• • • • • •

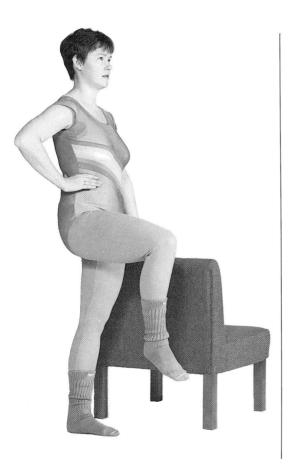

2 Raise the right knee upwards towards your chest. Repeat 4 times before changing legs. (If standing on one leg to lift your knee or bending forwards causes pain in your back, then avoid this exercise.)

ADDITIONAL EXERCISES FOR AFTER A CAESAREAN SECTION

If you have had a Caesarean section, include these exercises in addition to the other ones for the first few days. The breathing and coughing exercise helps to clear away any secretions in the lungs, and the leg exercises improve your circulation as you are likely to be less mobile.

Breathing and Coughing

Do some deep breathing with your main focus on the out breaths. As you breathe out, support your incision with your hands or a soft pillow. Keep your knees bent and instead of trying to give a proper cough, which will hurt, try huffing on the out breath.

Leg Exercises

Sit on the bed with your toes stretched out in front of you. Pull your toes up towards you and then point them away from you. Repeat this sequence about 20 times, moving briskly so that you really get the circulation going. You can move both feet in the same direction together or alternately, one up and one down.

Next, move your legs apart and circle your feet at the ankles, first in one direction and then the other.

Press the backs of your knees down into the bed and then release. This works the large thigh muscles and helps improve the circulation.

Bend one leg at a time, sliding your heel up the bed and then straighten that leg as you bend the other knee.

• • • • • •

MASSAGE

Massage can be another way of getting rid of backache caused by muscle tension. Massage improves the blood supply and tends to speed up the dispersal of waste products which are a cause of stiffness and soreness in the muscles. It can also help you to feel more relaxed and calm.

Encourage your partner to give you a massage at the end of a long and tiring day. You can always reciprocate when you are feeling less tired. Massage can be just as relaxing for the giver as it is for the receiver and can be a good way of expressing your love for each other, especially if you are not yet ready for full sexual intercourse.

It is a good idea to use something like plain vegetable oil or talcum powder on your hands to prevent friction. When you give a massage, avoid the bony areas as this can be very uncomfortable and try to relax your hands and mould to the area you are massaging. Pour a little oil onto the palm of your hand and use stroking movements to spread it over the skin.

Lavender, marjoram and rosemary are aromatherapy oils which are specifically for muscle stiffness and fatigue. They are rather expensive but you may feel like giving yourselves a treat and they will last a long time. Follow the instructions for dilution carefully as they must not be used undiluted.

> **❝In common with most of my close female friends who have recently had babies, my attitude to sex has changed quite dramatically since I had my daughter. I'm lucky to have a very understanding partner, but it does worry me a great deal that I might never feel the same way sexually again. Physically there is no problem, but I really couldn't be less interested — which is dreadful as I love my partner so much and we are much closer than ever in every way since we had the baby.❞**

Massage may be something you would like to try with your baby too. Babies usually love being massaged. It is probably best to use only a mild vegetable oil on her skin in case she is allergic to the stronger aromatherapy oils. (Instructions for baby massage are given on page 34.)

Neck and Back ☆

Find a comfortable position either lying face down on the bed or sitting at a table with your forehead resting on your hands on a pillow. Keep your head straight rather than turned to one side or the other as this puts unnecessary strain on the neck muscles. It is important for the person doing the massage to be relaxed and comfortable or any tension in them may transmit itself to you through their hands. Keep the wrists and fingers relaxed and use body weight to increase the pressure rather than the arm muscles alone.

Effleurage (this means stroke or glide)

When done as a light stroking movement in any direction on the body effleurage can be very soothing and relaxing. These are just two examples.

Place one hand on the top of each shoulder. Starting with the right hand, lightly stroke downwards on the right side towards the small of the back. When the right hand reaches the small of the back, start stroking down with the left hand at the same time replacing the right one back over the shoulder again ready to repeat the stroking action with that hand. Alternating the hands in this way ensures that there is always a hand in contact with the skin of the back, which feels very nice.

Another effleurage technique is a gliding, stroking movement using slightly deeper pressure to improve circulation. This is always done in one direction – from the extremities towards the heart (for example from the toes towards the hips). This helps to encourage the blood to flow back towards the heart.

Kneading

Kneading can be done with the palms of the hands or the finger tips and is a deep circular movement where the hand and the skin are moved together over the underlying muscles rather than just rubbing over the surface of the skin which can create uncomfortable friction. After a few circular movements in one area, the hands are gradually moved from one area to another so that the main bulky part of the muscle is eventually covered. This is particularly helpful in getting rid of tight little knots of muscle which tend to cause pain in the large upper back muscles in the shoulder and neck region.

Face Massage

It is very relaxing to have your face massaged, gently easing away the frown and worry lines. You can do most of the techniques described below for yourself, using fingertips rather than thumbs except where instructed to use thumbs, but it is definitely more relaxing to have someone else do it for you. Stroking, kneading and finger pressure are the most useful techniques to employ. Care needs to be taken to avoid dragging the delicate skin around the eyes. A moisturising cream is probably the

most appropriate as a lubricant for a face massage.

Use both thumbs and gradually stroke up from the bridge of the nose and out towards the edge of the eyebrows. With each stroke, move a little higher up the forehead away from the eyebrows.

Press gently and firmly in the centre of the forehead with both thumbs side by side. Hold for a few seconds and move a little higher before repeating the pressure.

Gently knead with the fingertips around the jaw line and try simple strokes across the chin.

....

WATCHPOINTS
● During massage, feedback to your partner about what feels right is very important. Is the pressure too hard or too light for example.

● It is important to keep parts of the body not being massaged covered to avoid getting cold.

● The person giving the massage must make sure he/she is in a comfortable position, avoiding any tension on the back, shoulders or arms. This will soon transmit itself to the person receiving the massage as well as not being good for the one giving the massage.

● Avoid dragging the skin or digging in with the fingers. Keep the hands as relaxed as possible and provide most of the pressure needed through the palms of the hands unless specifically doing thumb or finger kneading.

....

● ● ● ● ● ●

BABY MASSAGE

Massaging your baby should always be fun and enjoyable for you both. If she seems fractious, massage may soothe her but if it seems to make the situation worse, leave it until another time and try again.

You can use stroking and effleurage effectively on your baby's back and abdomen but because her limbs are so small, kneading the muscles of the arms and legs might be a little difficult. Use simple compression instead. Support the limb with one hand and encircle the limb with your other hand and gently squeeze. Hold for a few seconds and then release and move a little further up the limb until you have covered the whole area.

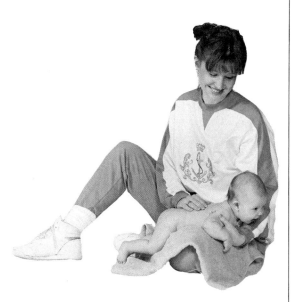

Lie your baby face down on a soft surface or across your lap. Place both hands on the top of her back near the shoulders, one on each side of her back bone. Gently draw your hands down towards her bottom in a firm stroking movement. Repeat 4–5 times. You can then try using one hand at a time. Always keep one hand in contact while you move the other one back to the starting position.

Abdomen

Keep your strokes light while massaging this area and watch your baby's responses as this is quite a sensitive area. Lie your baby on her back and gently stroke her tummy in a circular motion, in a clockwise direction. Start near the navel (tummy button) and gradually make your circles bigger (you should only do this massage when the navel has properly healed).

Arms and Shoulders

Lie your baby on her back and place your hands over the tops of her shoulders. Gently move both hands across her shoulders and down her arms towards her hands, encircling her arms with your whole hand. Move your hands one at a time back to the shoulders and start again.

Holding one of her hands in your hand, place your other hand around her upper arm and give a gentle squeeze, then release. Move your hand down a little further and squeeze again and release. Repeat these movements until you have reached her hand. With your thumb in her palm and your fingers on the back of her hand, gently knead her soft little hand, using a circular movement with your thumb and gently uncurling her fingers as you do so.

You could finish by playing 'Round and round the garden' (see right) with her. Then repeat the whole sequence on the other arm.

Legs

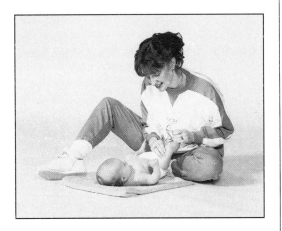

1 Lie your baby on her back. Using long firm gentle movements, stroke from the top of her thigh to her foot with first one hand, and then the other, always keeping one hand in contact. Repeat a number of times before changing legs.

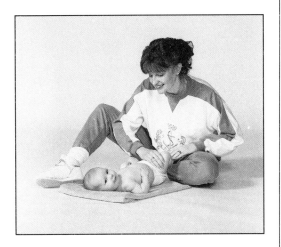

2 Lie your baby on her back and holding her ankle in one hand, place your other hand on the top of her thigh. Squeeze gently, encircling her thigh with one hand and then releasing the pressure before moving down the leg a little. Continue until you reach her foot and then change to the other leg.

Face

Although you may find it very relaxing to have your face massaged, most babies don't like it and won't relax and stay still. If you feel like trying it, then it's probably best to avoid covering the eyes or mouth with your hands and just concentrate on stroking her forehead and head, using your finger tips or the palms of your hands. A gentle stroking movement is all that you need.

Round and Round the Garden

As you say the words, **round and round the garden like a teddy bear,** draw little circles in her palm with one of your fingers. Then make two stepping movements with your fingers as you say
One step, two step, and then run your fingers up her arm and tickle her under the armpit as you say **and tickle her under there.**

Your body after six weeks

About 6–8 weeks after the birth, you will see your midwife, GP or consultant for a postnatal checkup to make sure that you have fully recovered from the birth. In many cases, women are given time to discuss, with the doctor, their feelings about all aspects of the birth and how it was managed, as well as talking about any postnatal health issues. Unfortunately, for some women it is a rather quick examination with little chance for discussion. This just helps to re-inforce the feeling some women experience, that now they are no longer pregnant, the baby's health is far more important as far as the GP is concerned than their own.

This visit should be a good opportunity for you to discuss contraception as well as anything about your health or the baby that may be worrying you. It might be helpful to make a list of the things you wish to discuss and try to make a specific appointment rather than attend a busy drop-in surgery.

You will probably be given an internal examination and a cervical smear test at the same time. If you are having any problems such as pain on sexual intercourse, stress incontinence or if you are anxious that your abdominal muscles don't seem to be returning to normal as quickly as you thought they would, this is the time to talk to the midwife or doctor about it. It is important to be honest about how you are really feeling especially if you feel worn out and not interested in much. Don't try to pretend that everything is wonderful if it isn't. (See page 94 for more information about postnatal depression.)

If you had a Caesarean section, you should be allowed to fully discuss the reasons why the Caesarean was necessary and any problems you may have about your recovery.

• • • • • •

EXERCISING AFTER SIX WEEKS

If you exercise regularly during the first few weeks, you should be feeling much stronger and have more energy by the time you reach the six-week stage. You can then move on to a fuller exercise programme that will continue to improve your fitness. Some women feel able to move on to these exercises before six weeks but there are certain guidelines you should follow. If you are sure your rectus abdominus muscles have come together again to approximately two finger width or less and you can comfortably do about 15 of the curl-ups on page 26 for a few consecutive days, you are ready to move on. Watch your abdomen when you do the curl-ups. If the muscles are bulging or shaking then the exercise is too strong. RETURN TO THE LESS STRENUOUS ONES for a little longer.

If you have had a Caesarean section then you should continue to do the less difficult exercises until about 10–12 weeks after the operation.

Included in this exercise programme are a number of exercises you would find in an exercise-to-music class such as warm-up and stretch exercises, low impact aerobic exercises, muscular strength and endurance and cool-down exercises. You may choose to do the exercises to music that you like. If so, it is most important that you choose carefully. Music with a definite beat can help encourage you to move, but beware of a tempo that encourages you to move at a speed which feels uncomfortably fast. The music should never dictate how you do the exercise but rather should motivate you and enhance the exercise.

The quality of the movement depends on doing it at the correct speed for you and is important in ensuring that you get the most out of the exercises and avoid injury. It is possible to use a piece of music that may seem fast if you count and move at half the speed i.e. 1 – AND – 2 – AND instead of 1,2,1,2.

Music for the warm-up and cool-down should be rhythmical with a good beat. For muscular strength and endurance it should be much slower. Don't choose music that encourages you to do curl-ups, for example, at a speed which does not allow enough time for you to rest your head and neck in between each curl-up. For the aerobic section, choose the sort of cheerful music that would get you walking at a brisk pace or makes you feel like dancing. Stretching should always be done smoothly and slowly without bouncing or jerking and any music you choose for that section should reflect that. At the end of the book, some suggestions have been made of the type of music which is appropriate for each section but this is purely as a guide.

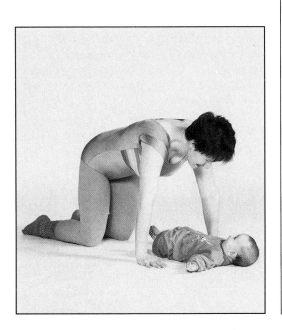

EXERCISES WITH YOUR BABY

A number of the exercises in this programme can be safely performed together with your baby. In some exercises, holding her will give your muscles added resistance and make you work harder. In others, she may be lying on the floor beside you, just watching you exercising. Either way she will probably enjoy the movement and the closeness.

Check that you are able to support her well while still being able to perform your exercises correctly and without strain.

The exercises are all described to show you the correct way to perform them on your own. In some of the photographs you will see a mother doing the exercise while holding the baby. Where necessary, extra instructions are given.

Decide day to day, depending on how you and your baby are feeling, whether or not to include her in your exercise session. You may prefer to concentrate on your exercises while she is asleep, or being looked after by someone else, or you may choose to use your exercise session as a time when you can enjoy your baby's company and get to know her better. If you are both feeling relaxed and happy, she should enjoy being held close to you while you move or she may just like lying beside you watching you move.

However, if she is very irritable and fractious and you find yourself becoming frustrated at your attempts to exercise, it is probably best to abandon the exercise session for the time being and try again at a different time. You could always go for a brisk walk with the pram instead. This should have the dual benefit of calming down the baby as well as building up your aerobic fitness. You could then return to the other kinds of exercises later in the day.

• • • • • •

THE BENEFITS OF EXERCISE

Taking regular exercise can bring with it many benefits to health. These include:

• Improvement in the heart and lungs, which in the long term reduces the risk of coronary heart disease.

• A most effective means of weight control when combined with monitoring your calorie intake.

• Joining an exercise class is a good way of meeting other people.

• It can improve your body shape by toning flabby muscles and reducing fat stores and give you a feeling of well-being.

• It can be a good way of coping with stress induced tension.

• Exercise can help reduce some of the effects of ageing.

• It can reduce or help prevent the effects of certain conditions like high blood pressure (a major risk factor relating to heart disease), diabetes mellitus and osteoporosis (a condition very common in post menopausal women where the bones become less dense, making them more prone to breaking).

In one four-year study of two groups of women in America (see References on page 142), one group exercising and the other not, researchers found that the women in the exercise group in some cases increased their bone mineral content and certainly lost far less of their bone mineral content than the women in the non-exercise group. The non-exercisers also decreased in fitness and gained weight in comparison.

Many people think that to be really fit you have to spend hours a week jogging, lifting heavy weights in a gym or taking part in hectic aerobics classes dressed in the latest fashionable leotards. This book shows you how to get the benefits of exercise with a minimum of effort in your own home. It may also encourage you to then go out and find the sort of exercise activity that you will enjoy so that you can keep up the good work started here.

Physical fitness includes a number of different components such as Suppleness, Muscular Strength and Endurance, Stamina or Cardiovascular fitness (sometimes known as the 3 S's) and Balance and Co-ordination. To be really fit you should work on all these elements to ensure a good balance. Certain activities work on one main element only and you would then need to take up a different activity to improve the other areas of fitness. For example, yoga develops suppleness but doesn't do much for your stamina; weight training develops muscular strength but doesn't necessarily improve suppleness. Swimming is one activity that rates highly for all three S's.

Walking is a very good way of improving and maintaining fitness providing you follow a few basic guidelines. Walking at an average pace is a very efficient form of exercise and therefore doesn't burn up many calories. To improve fitness and burn up more calories, you need to walk at a brisk enough pace to make you feel a bit puffed.

It also needs to be for long enough and often enough to be effective. A brisk walk to the shops for 5 minutes with the pram is not enough. You need to walk for at least 15 –30 minutes about 3–5 times a week if you want to improve your fitness and help to keep your weight down. Even this level of exercise is not sufficient to prevent the post- menopausal bone loss so you will need to do some other form of exercise as well.

> **❝The classes were great. It's already got my husband and I exercising at home.❞**

Walking up a hill, especially with a pram, will increase the amount of work your muscles and heart have to do. If you have a hill to climb to reach the local shops, be grateful for the good it's doing you.

It is important that any exercise you do, whether it's a brisk walk or a time set aside for special exercises, should not be a boring chore done when you don't really feel like it. If it becomes a chore, you will probably feel worn out by the time you have finished rather than feeling relaxed and full of energy. Choose your time carefully and this way you will really benefit from the feelings of well being that can be gained from exercising.

SAFETY IN EXERCISE

Any exercise programme, no matter how carefully designed, has the potential for causing injury. If you know what the common mistakes are, you can do your best to avoid them and keep your exercising as safe as possible.

People who are more prone to injury are those who:
- Have very poor flexibility.
- Are very overweight.
- Have poor muscle tone.
- Have not done any exercise for a long time.

Practical Ideas for Safe Exercising

Exercises should never cause pain, dizziness, tightness in the chest or difficulty in breathing. If they do you should STOP. If you feel any mild discomfort, it may be due to muscles unused to work or the use of an incorrect starting position. Check your position and read the instructions carefully. If the exercise still causes you pain, check it out with your GP.

Never exercise when unwell or recovering from illness. Allow at least 2 days for recovery after something like a bout of 'flu.

If you really feel worn out or have persistent muscle aches and pains or if your pulse rates fails to return to its normal resting rate for a long time after finishing your exercise session you have probably overdone it and should modify what you do the next time. (For a full explanation about pulse rates, see the aerobic section, page 55.)

Doing a vigorous exercise session every day of the week makes you more prone to overuse injuries – 3–5 times a week is all that is necessary to keep you fit.

Wear loose comfortable clothing that allows your body to breathe. Leotards and tights are not really necessary – they have been used in the photographs so that you can clearly see the movements. Layers of clothes, which can be removed and replaced during and after exercise are a good idea. Your shoes should be non-slip with soft soles and well-cushioned heels, especially for aerobic work. Do not do aerobic exercises with bare feet.

Don't have the temperature in the room where you are exercising too hot or too cold. Make sure that there are no obstacles or doors to bump into or slippery floor surfaces. Check what your toddler is up to when you are exercising; you can do the exercises together or you can settle him down nearby with some toys.

After the birth, many women have discomfort in their coccyx. If liked, for the floor exercises, lie on a blanket, towel or exercise mat to protect your spine when doing exercises like curl-ups and curl-downs. Stop any exercises which cause pain.

Always build-up and slow-down the intensity of the exercises gradually.

Don't exercise within 2 hours of eating a big meal.

Lastly, don't forget to SMILE. Think of all the benefits: exercising should be enjoyable – not a chore.

• • • • • •

SAFETY GUIDELINES

Remember the basic posture when doing all standing exercises:

THINK TALL

ABDOMEN PULLED IN AND PELVIS TUCKED UNDER

SHOULDERS PRESSED BACK AND DOWN

KNEES SOFT AND NOT LOCKED BACK

CHIN IN AND NECK LONG

BREATHE NORMALLY

When doing any exercise that involves bending your knees, make sure that your knees are directly over your toes to avoid straining the ligaments on the inside of your knees and ankles.

When doing curl-ups, always have your knees bent with your feet flat on the floor and your abdominal muscles firmly contracted to keep your back flat on the floor. When progressing to the stronger exercise with hands beside the head, make sure that your fingers are spread out beside your ears. DO NOT clasp your hands behind your head as this can pull on your neck.

When doing any exercises on all-fours, keep the abdomen pulled in and keep your back flat.

When doing any head and neck exercises, keep the movements slow and smooth.

EXERCISES TO AVOID

DON'T drop your head back too far to look up at the ceiling. This puts a lot of strain on the neck joints.

AVOID deep knee bends as this puts too much strain around the knee joint. Keep the thigh parallel with the floor.

AVOID bouncy, jerky movements when trying to increase your range of movement in the suppleness exercises. They simply bring in the stretch reflex and do not increase the range of movement at all; for example, toe touches with straight legs force the knees to overextend and can put a lot of strain on the lower back. It will also cause the muscles on the backs of your thighs to tighten to stop you causing any damage to your knees and back. This exercise is often portrayed in the mistaken belief that it will improve the stretch in the back of the thighs.

NEVER lift both legs in the air when lying flat on your back. This puts a great strain on the back, especially if you have weakened abdominal muscles.

AVOID doing sit ups with your legs straight as this is also likely to strain the back. Always have your knees bent.

FIRST AID

If you follow the safety precautions and guidelines listed on the previous pages you should not have any first aid problems. However, if you do have problems, knowing what to do immediately can lessen any tissue damage and speed up the healing process.

Any injury that does not improve quickly with the following first aid treatment, or is causing you problems, should be seen by a doctor or physiotherapist without delay.

Whether the injury is a muscle strain or tear, a direct knock to a limb, or a sprain in the ligaments surrounding and supporting a joint, such as a twisted ankle, the results are all very similar. There is usually pain followed by swelling and then bruising in the immediate area of the injury. This leads to immobility of the limb and the longer that persists the more chance there is of joint stiffness and some muscle weakness developing. If you can keep the swelling and bruising to a minimum, you will help reduce the pain and make the recovery that much faster. For most minor limb injuries the most effective treatment is a combination of rest, ice, compression and elevation.

REST means not using the limb for a day or two while healing takes place. ICE acts by relieving pain and reducing the blood flow to the area which in turn reduces the tendency for the injured limb to swell. COMPRESSION is applied to the affected part by means of a crêpe or elastic bandage. ELEVATION is important for areas like the ankle or hand, which will swell due to the effects of gravity if allowed to hang down. Raising the leg up on a stool or putting the arm in a sling will reduce the blood flow and therefore reduce the swelling and the pain.

66 *Beware of too high expectations. Exercise to your own level.* **99**

EXERCISING WITH A DISABILITY

There are many different forms of disability, ranging from physical and mental conditions to visual and hearing impairment. Within each category of disability there are a wide range of conditions, each one varying in its effects. Visual impairment, for example, ranges from complete loss of vision to partial sight. A large percentage of those people who are registered blind, are affected by severe visual problems rather than total blindness. Only about 5% have no perception of light at all.

There are many types of physical disability resulting from illness, injury or congenital abnormalities. For example paralysis may be caused by a spinal injury, cerebral palsy or multiple sclerosis. The extent of the muscles affected and the type of paralysis will vary tremendously. It is not possible in a book like this to give specific adaptations of exercises for each type of disability; however, it is possible to give some general guidelines about exercising with a disability.

If you have a disability, you may find that you are able to do many of the exercises in this programme just as they are described. There will be other exercises that you cannot manage at all, and some where you will need to adapt the starting position so that, for example, you are sitting instead of standing. The particular type of disability and how much it affects you, will determine which exercises you are able to do. You will know what your limitations are. Look at the exercises and decide which ones might be the right ones for you. If you have any difficulties deciding, ask to speak to an obstetric physiotherapist and discuss with her what you can do and how to adapt the exercise programme for you. If you have difficulties with muscle spasms, it may be better to avoid certain exercises but there may be possible alternatives.

The most important exercises for women after having a baby are starred. If you can't manage all the exercises, concentrate on these starred ones. The basic principles of exercising remain the same. Do as much as you feel able to do and let your body guide you as to how many you do or for how long you exercise. Any increase over and above your normal daily activity levels will be beneficial. To avoid fatigue, doing a few short bouts of exercises may be better than one long session.

It is possible to do aerobic exercises, which will get your heart and lungs working, while sitting in a chair. If you have movement in your arms, you can do the arm circling, side bends and head trunk and shoulder rotation exercises.

If you have problems with your balance and you need to support yourself with one hand while moving the other arm, you can do all those exercises with one arm at a time while holding onto some support.

Alternate clapping of your hands together above your head, then onto your knees is a good exercise if you can move both arms together. Don't hold both arms above your head for long periods as this will cause muscle fatigue in your shoulders and can cause your blood pressure to go up. It is better to keep them moving rhythmically.

If you can move your legs but find standing difficult because of balance, the following leg exercises can be done in a sitting position.

Straighten first one leg out in front of you and then bend it and replace the foot on the floor. Repeat with the other leg. Alternate until you have done 6–8 on each side. You could then add in your arms, stretching one above your head as you straighten the opposite leg.

Sit with your knees bent and your thighs well supported. Keeping your knee bent, lift first your right thigh up off the chair and then replace your right foot flat on the floor. Repeat with the other leg. Continue to alternate legs as if you were marking time on the spot. This will certainly get your circulation going and raise your pulse.

You may not be able to raise your pulse

66 Don't think you shouldn't do any exercises at all just because you can't manage to do all of them.99

level into your training zone (see page 56) but any increase will be beneficial. If you find that your pulse has increased quite considerably, especially if it is near the top of your training zone you will need to tone down the exercises a little. Make sure you are breathing calmly, don't move so quickly and bring the arms down. You could try stretching them out in front of you instead of above your head.

Remember when you first start exercising your aim should be to get your pulse into your lower training zone. If you are taking any medication that has an effect on your pulse rate, you will need to use your perceived exertion as described on page 55 rather than your pulse rate as a guide to tell you if you are working at an effective and safe level.

If you spend a large part of the day sitting in a wheelchair you may feel that you are very restricted in what you can do in the way of exercise. You may feel that if you can't manage to exercise on your own, it is all too much of an effort.

If you can get someone to help you out of the chair and onto the floor or a firm bed and do some of the exercises with you, it will benefit you in a number of ways. It will give you a chance to stretch out some of the muscles and joints which tend to shorten and stiffen up when kept in one position all day long. Lying on your front for a period each day will help to avoid stiff hips and knee joints and by lifting your head a few times while lying in that position, you will be exercising your back muscles.

Rolling over from your back to your front will also be very good abdominal exercise and if you can get someone to bend your knees and support them in that position while you lift your head and shoulders you will strengthen your abdominal muscles.

You and your baby will probably also enjoy the different perspective of being able to lie down and exercise together. An older child can also join in with the exercises.

Sitting in your wheelchair and reaching behind you to get something off a table or shelf, rather than swinging the chair round to face the table or shelf first, is very good exercise for suppleness of the spine and the twisting action will work your oblique abdominal muscles.

If you have a visual impairment, you will not be able to see the photographs so you will need someone to describe the exercise to you initially so that you get the positions and actions correct. You could tape record someone reading the exercises. You might find it helpful to do the exercises together with a friend. Some of the exercises in the aerobic section, can be done with 2 people holding hands together, for example when doing the backwards and forwards walking. In exercise classes participants are occasionally encouraged to form a circle and exercise together to add to the enjoyment. This may or may not work for you. If holding hands with someone tends to knock you off balance, then you can do the same exercise marking time on one spot without travelling in a forwards or backwards direction. It will be just as effective. If you need support, hold onto a chair back.

If you have a hearing impairment which prevents you listening to music, you can perform the exercises just as well at your own pace. You can count your own rhythm. As mentioned earlier, music isn't always an advantage as it can sometimes make people move too quickly or too slowly. Use your pulse rate, as well as how you are feeling, to check whether you are moving briskly enough in the aerobic section. The other exercises in the programme should be easy enough to follow using a combination of the written explanation and the photographs. Avoid exercises which put too much strain on your

joints, such as knee-bends and press-ups, if you have stiff and painful joints due to arthritis. Concentrate on improving the strength of your pelvic floor and abdominal muscles and keeping your joints mobile by doing some of the suppleness exercises. If you can manage it, do rhythmical arm swinging movements and knee lifts in a sitting position, as this will improve both your stamina and suppleness. Swimming is a very good way of improving suppleness, strength and stamina without putting undue strain on any joints because the buoyancy of the water supports your body weight. However, there will be times when your joints are inflamed and painful when rest is more important than exercise. During these times, concentrate on practising your relaxation techniques in different positions until you find the most comfortable ones for you.

As you are coping with a disability as well as the physical demands of looking after a young baby, you may find that you get extremely tired. Make time to relax and restore some energy during the day, tackling chores and activities in short spells with frequent rest periods. It may seem as if you will never fit in anything that way but you will be surprised at how much better and more quickly you are able to tackle things when well rested.

WARM-UP AND STRETCH SECTION

WARM-UP

The warm-up is an important part of any exercise programme and its aim is to prepare the body for exercise and help to prevent muscle fatigue and injury, such as sprains and muscle tears.

Never think of it as a waste of time or energy and don't skimp it if you are short of time. It should always include some rhythmic activity which gradually increases in intensity and should be of sufficient intensity to work up a light sweat by the time you have finished. The benefits include:

• A gradual increase in the body temperature which will improve the speed at which energy is released to the muscles.

• An improvement in the blood supply to the muscles and joints which in turn improves their oxygen supply.

• A reduction in the risk of injury by warming-up cold muscles.

• A gradual preparation of the heart and lungs for more strenuous exercises such as those in the aerobic section.

The warm-up should also include some stretching, especially of the large muscles which will be used in the aerobic and strength sections of the exercise programme. Warmed-up muscles will stretch better than cold ones and will be less prone to injury. See page 51 for stretches.

Knee Bends and Shoulder Shrugs

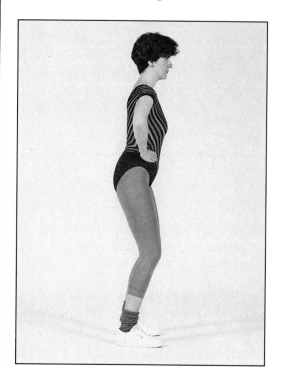

Stand with feet apart, toes very slightly turned out, weight evenly on both feet and knees slightly bent. Bottom tucked under and tummy pulled in. Hands on hips.
Bend your knees, keeping knees over toes and working the thigh muscles. Don't bend and stretch too fast. Bend for 2 beats of the music and straighten for 2 beats. Repeat 4 times. Now transfer your weight from one foot to another as you straighten up after each knee bend, pointing the toe of the straight leg out to one side as you do so. Keep your shoulders level. Repeat 4 times to each foot. Finally, add shoulder shrugs up and down as you transfer the weight from foot to foot. Repeat 4 times to each side. Keep breathing smoothly throughout the exercise.

• • • • • •

Arm Circles

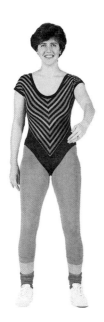

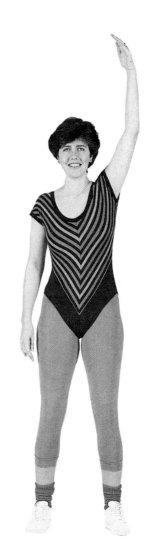

1 Stand with feet apart, toes very slightly turned out, weight evenly on both feet and knees slightly bent. Make sure your bottom is tucked under and tummy pulled in. Circle your left arm up and forwards.

WATCHPOINTS
- If you are breastfeeding you will need to wear good breast pads inside your bra while you are exercising, otherwise you will find that you leak, especially when moving your arms around a lot.
- Keep the arms close the ears.
- Don't arch your back to compensate for stiff shoulders.
- Check that arms are circling in a forward direction.
- Breathe rhythmically throughout the exercise.

2 Bring your arm up past your left ear, bending your knees as the arm comes down past your knees and straightening them as the arm swings upwards. Return to your start position and repeat 4 times with the left arm. Change arms and repeat exercise with the right arm 4 times.

• • • • •

Pelvic Tilt and Circles

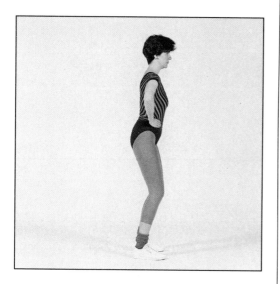

1 Stand with feet hip-width apart, knees slightly bent, bottom tucked under, tummy and pelvic floor muscles pulled in.

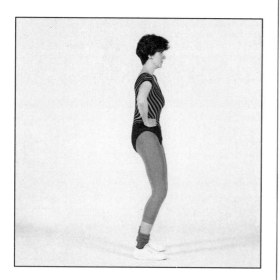

2 Tip the pelvis forwards, arching the back very slightly and then tuck the pelvis under, tightening the buttocks. Continue in a rocking movement. Repeat 4 times.

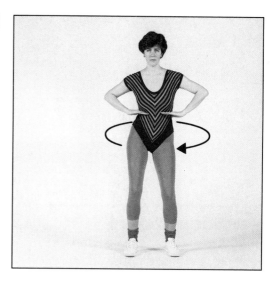

3 Now draw a large circle with your hips, left, forwards, right and back. Repeat twice in one direction, making sure you move your hips not your knees. Change and repeat twice in the other direction.

....

WATCHPOINTS
● Keep the range of movements small and don't over-emphasise the arching of the back.
● Keep the movements slow and rhythmical.
● Concentrate on the feel of tucking the pelvis under and pulling in the abdominal muscles.
● When doing all your exercise programme, remember to keep the pelvis tucked under in this way and the abdominals pulled in as there will be a tendency to revert back to the forward tilting, flabby tummy posture of pregnancy.

....

Walking Forwards and Back

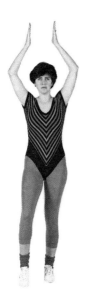

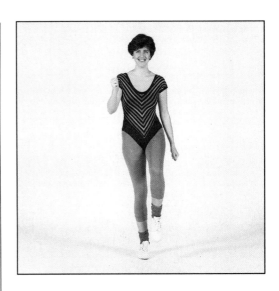

1 Stand as for pelvic tilt and circles. Walk forwards for 4 steps, clapping your hands together above your head on the last step, i.e. forwards-2-3-clap.

3 March on the spot for 8 counts, swinging the arms briskly by your side.

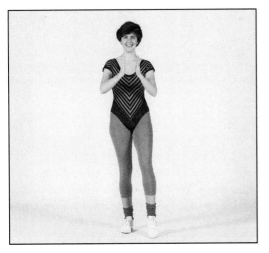

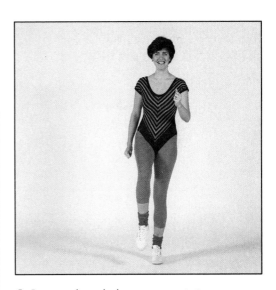

4 Repeat the whole sequence twice.

2 Change direction by walking backwards for 4 steps, clapping your hands together on the last step, backwards-2-3-clap.

• • • • • •

Side Bends

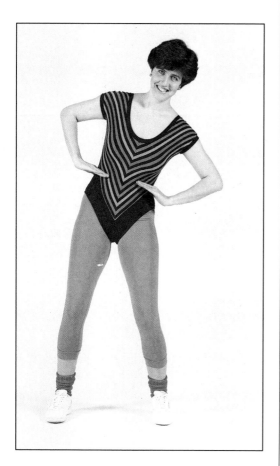

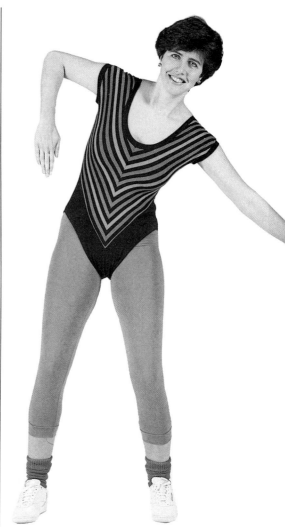

1 Stand with feet hip-width apart, knees soft, pelvis tucked under and tummy and pelvic floor muscles pulled in. Hand on hips. Bend sideways towards your left side.

WATCHPOINT
● Be careful not to lean forward or back but bend directly sideways without bouncing.

2 Reach out with the left arm and gently bend the right one up under your right armpit. Return to the centre, stretching your arms out in front at shoulder height as you do so. Breathe out as you bend and in as you straighten up in the centre. Repeat, bending to the other side, then return to the centre. Repeat the whole exercise 4 times to each side.

Head, Trunk and Shoulder Rotations

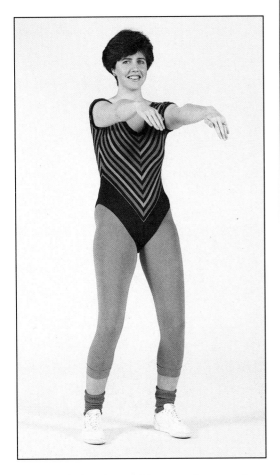

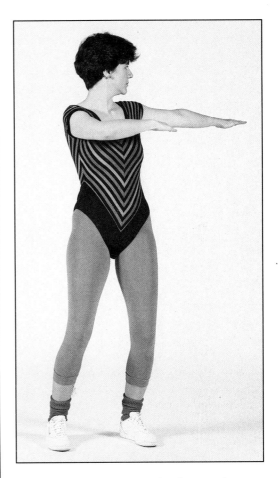

Stand with feet hip-width apart, knees soft, pelvis tucked under and tummy and pelvic floor muscles pulled in. Stretch out your arms in front at shoulder height.

Keeping your hips facing the front, with tummy pulled in and bottom tucked under, swivel from the waist to look behind you. Return to face the front. Breathe out as you swivel round and in as you return to the centre. Keep your eyes on the fingers of the leading hand. Relax the trailing arm across your chest.

Knee Lifts

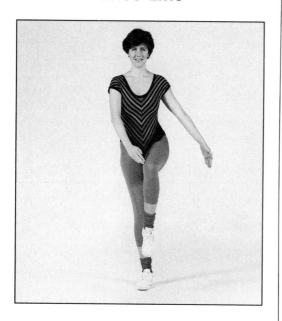

Stand with feet hip-width apart, weight evenly distributed, knees slightly bent and your hands on your hips. Raise one knee in front of you to about hip height and touch your knee with the fingertips of the opposite hand, swinging your other hand out to your side. Replace that foot on the ground and repeat the exercise with the other leg. Repeat 4 times on each side.

WATCHPOINT
● Transferring your weight from foot to foot with a knee bent like this may cause pain if you have any problems with your sacro-iliac joint. If so, try just pointing alternate toes in front of you as you step from foot to foot and stretch the opposite arm down in front of you towards the knee.

Lunges

Stand with feet apart, slightly wider than your hips and turned out slightly, keeping your knees over your toes. Hands on hips, bottom tucked under and tummy pulled in. Bend your left knee and transfer all your weight over that leg. Transfer across to the other side smoothly and rhythmically. Repeat 4 times. Repeat the lunges, this time, taking the arms DOWN towards the opposite knee each time. Repeat 4 times to each side.

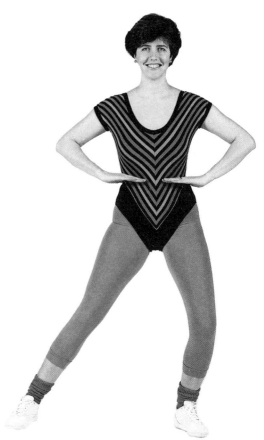

STRETCH SECTION

The aim of these stretch exercises is to help warm-up your muscles so that they will stretch easily as you work through your exercise programme.

When a muscle is stretched, the stretch reflex comes into play. This makes the muscle contract to prevent it from being overstretched and so protects the joints from damage. If you perform the stretch too quickly in a bouncy sort of movement, you are much more likely to cause injury to that muscle. If you perform the stretch in a smooth and controlled way, holding it for about 6–8 seconds, the stretch reflex is gradually overcome and the muscle will then be able to stretch safely and effectively.

Start with the gastrocnemius stretch and work through them in order.

Gastrocnemius (Calf Muscle) Stretch

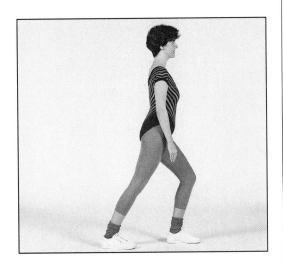

Stand with feet hip-width apart. Stretch the right leg out behind you at least 30 cm (12 inches) behind the left foot with the toes of both feet facing straight forwards. Keep your pelvis tucked under to avoid arching your back. Keeping the right leg straight and the left knee bent, lean forward slightly with your weight over the left leg until you feel a stretch at the back of the right calf. (Make sure that the front knee is directly over the toes so that the shin bone is vertical from the ground.) Keep the right heel on the ground. Hold for a few seconds.

Soleus (Calf Muscle) Stretch

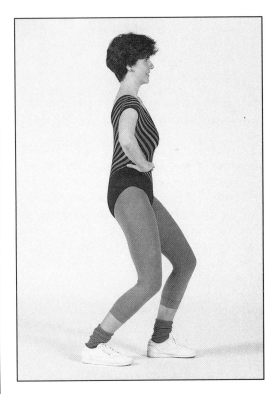

Straighten up and bring the right foot in a few inches towards the left. Transfer your weight over the right foot, bending the knee slightly, and straighten the left leg out in front of you. Keep your pelvis tucked under to avoid arching your back. You should now feel a stretch lower down in the right calf. Hold the position for a few seconds.

Hamstring (Muscle on the Back of the Thigh) Stretch

Now lean forwards from the hips with your hands resting on the right thigh above the knee. Keep the left leg straight and feel the stretch in the back of your left thigh. Hold for a few seconds and then straighten up and change legs. Repeat all 3 stretches on the other side.

....

WATCHPOINT
- During the hamstring stretch don't press on the actual knee joint.
....

Quadriceps (the Muscles on the Front of the Thigh) Stretch

Stand with feet hip-width apart, bend your right leg up behind you and grasp your right ankle with your right hand. Keeping both knees together and your pelvis tucked in, ease the right thigh as far behind you as you can and you should feel the stretch down the front of the right thigh. Hold for a few seconds and repeat with the left leg. (Hold onto a chair or the wall with the other hand if you find it difficult to balance on one foot.)
....

WATCHPOINTS
- Hold around the ankle and not the toes to avoid straining the ankle joint.
- Keep the bent knee close to the knee of the standing leg. If you allow it to drift out to the side you don't get such a good stretch down the front of the thigh.
- Keep your bottom tucked under and don't allow your back to arch.
....

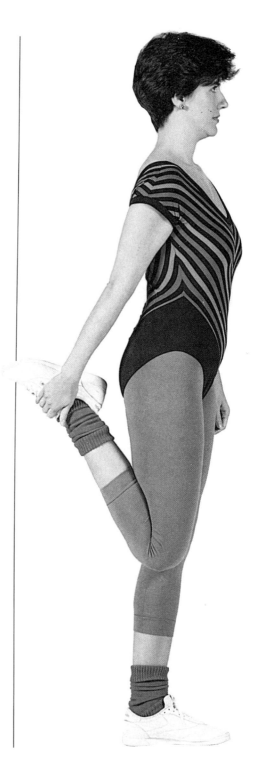

Triceps (the Muscle on the Back of the Upper Arm) Stretch

Pectoral (the Muscle Across the Front of the Chest) Stretch

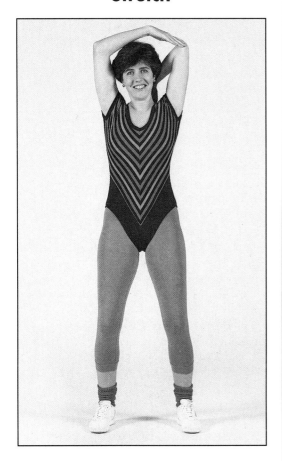

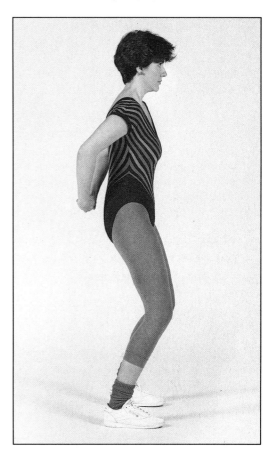

Stand with feet hip-width apart and knees soft, tummy pulled in and pelvis tucked under. Stretch your left arm above your head, close to your left ear, then drop the hand down behind your head. Take your right hand across and, clasping the left elbow, pull it across towards the right. Feel the stretch down the back of your left arm. Do not poke your head forward or arch your back. Hold for a few seconds and repeat the stretch with the other arm.

Stand with feet hip-width apart and knees soft, tummy pulled in and pelvis tucked under. Clasp both hands behind your back and pull them up and back as far as you comfortably can. You should feel a stretch in the muscles across the front of your chest. Avoid locking out the elbow joints. If your breasts are painful, avoid this exercise for the time being.

• • • • • •   • • • • • •

AEROBIC OR STAMINA SECTION

The aim of this section is to improve fitness in the cardiovascular system (the heart, lungs and blood vessels). This is an essential part of fitness, which should not be neglected at this very busy time in your life. Cardiovascular fitness is an important aspect in reducing the risk of coronary heart disease, a disease strongly linked to lifestyle. We are all to some extent at risk of this disease which currently kills about 500 people a day in Britain. Women are protected to a certain degree, by their hormones but after the menopause are as much at risk as men of the same age. Smoking, a high fat and high sugar diet, high blood pressure, lack of exercise and stress are all major contributing factors. However, armed with the correct information and motivation, we can alter these factors if we choose to.

The word Aerobics is much misused these days and it generally conjures up images of the kind of hectic exercise classes where people jump and jog to the point of near exhaustion. The term AEROBIC means 'with oxygen' and refers to the type of activity during which the muscles of the body convert stored fuel into energy in the presence of oxygen. Muscles are capable of producing energy ANAEROBICALLY (without oxygen) but this tends to be a less efficient way to mobilise the required energy. It results in a rapid build up of waste products (mainly lactic acid) which limits the length of time the muscle can go on working efficiently (to about 40 seconds) and tends to cause muscle cramps and stiffness. A hundred metre sprint is almost entirely anaerobic exercise.

Running for a bus would leave most unfit people with aching muscles and gasping for air as their muscles ran out of sufficient oxygen. For an activity to continue for any length of time, sufficient oxygen is required. The heart, lungs and blood vessels are mainly responsible for delivering that oxygen to the working muscles.

Oxygen is extracted from the air in the lungs and transported via the blood vessels to all parts of the body, pumped by the heart. The heart is approximately the size of a clenched fist and is made of muscle. Like all muscles, it responds to exercise by becoming larger, stronger and more efficient. The amount of blood pumped out around the body with each heart beat is known as the Stroke Volume and this will vary depending on whether you are resting or active. The Heart Rate (the number of times the heart beats per minute) multiplied by the Stroke Volume amounts to the Cardiac Output i.e. the total amount of blood pumped in a minute.

Aerobic exercise is the way to improve cardiovascular fitness. With regular aerobic exercise, the heart muscle becomes stronger and the Stroke Volume increases so that with each heart beat the stronger heart is able to pump out more blood. The Heart Rate can therefore be reduced while still providing the same Cardiac Output. This means that the heart has to do less work for the same outcome and in the long term this is beneficial.

For aerobic or stamina exercise to be effective in training your heart, you have to work with your heart rate above a certain minimum level, and to be safe you need to work with it below a maximum level. Between these two levels is your safe and effective personal training zone (see page 56 for how to calculate your own).

Your heart rate can be monitored by taking your pulse. The pulse rate can be affected by all sorts of things, such as exercise, stress, caffeine or illness and it varies throughout the day, but it can be a useful way of monitoring whether or not you are exercising at the right level for you.

PULSE TAKING

Pulse rate is measured in beats per minute. You can count the beats for a full 15 seconds and multiply the number by four. It is important to remember to count your first beat as NOUGHT, 1, 2, 3 etc. This will give you your pulse rate for a minute.

Radial pulse: Place three fingers around your wrist on the thumb side and just above the skin crease. Press firmly and you should feel something pulsing beneath your fingertips. Don't use the thumb of the other hand to feel for your pulse as there is a pulse in your thumb and this will only cause confusion. Don't press too hard or you will block off some of the blood passing through the artery that you are trying to feel.

Carotid pulse: An alternative place to feel for your pulse is in the neck. Just below the angle of your jaw and directly below the ear lobe press inwards and upwards to the side of the Adam's apple and you should feel a pulse.

Resting pulse: Your resting pulse is your pulse rate when you have been resting for a long period. For example, if you took your pulse rate first thing in the morning when you woke up this would be your resting pulse. It would not be an accurate reading if you had just had a cup of tea or coffee or if you were still shaking from the shrill sound of the alarm clock startling you out of your peaceful sleep.

Start pulse: This is the pulse you take before you start exercising. It is a good guideline because if your pulse is already raised for some reason, you know not to work too hard or you may exceed your safe training zone.

Working pulse: This is the pulse you take within 10 seconds of finishing the exercise session. This gives you a measure of whether or not you were working at the right level for you. (You can of course take your pulse during the exercise session if you wish. This is useful when you first start an exercise programme until you get the feel of the exercises).

Recovery pulse: This is the pulse you take after you have finished exercising to see how quickly your heart rate recovers. Get into the habit of always taking your pulse at a specific point in your exercise programme (for example after the stretches) or about 90 seconds after you stop exercising. It is not an accurate guide to improving fitness if you sometimes take your recovery pulse 90 seconds after finishing and the next time 4 minutes after finishing.

As you get fitter you should be able to see some improvement. The fitter you are the more rapidly your heart rate will return to normal. As you get used to this type of exercise, you will find that you begin to recognise how your body feels when you are working at the appropriate heart rate level. (This is known as perceived exertion). You can then rely on this when doing any sort of exercise without always having to stop and take your pulse.

The following are appropriate symptoms to be experiencing while doing aerobic exercises.

● Increased breathing rate but still able to carry on a conversation.
● Feeling warm.
● Sweating slightly.
● Feeling that your muscles are working harder than usual.

The following are inappropriate symptoms that suggest you are exercising too hard and need to slow down and stop:
● Breathlessness to the point of being speechless.
● Very profuse sweating or cold sweat.
● Chest or leg pain.
● Dizziness or feeling faint.
● Nausea or vomiting.
● Heart pounding.

It is very important to remember that you should NEVER SUDDENLY STOP and stand still when you have been working your body hard during aerobic-type exercises.

Whether coming to the end of a regular exercise session or because you can feel the need to stop if it gets to be too much and you are starting to tire, you should always keep your legs moving gently until your pulse rate has come back down to a more normal level.

If you don't do this, a large amount of blood will pool down in the veins in your legs, and your heart, which is beating at a much faster rate, will suddenly find that it does not have the right amount of blood to pump around the body and, particularly, up to the brain. This could place unnecessary strain on the heart, as well as making you feel very dizzy. Marking time on the spot or just walking round slowly is sufficient to keep the blood circulating to all parts of the body.

PERSONAL PULSE RANGE

Heart rate is age related and decreases by approximately one beat per minute for each year of adult life. This needs to be taken into consideration when working out your own personal training zone for aerobic exercise. By subtracting your own age from the maximum figure of 200 you have a built-in safety factor when working out your own safe training zone.

CALCULATING YOUR OWN PERSONAL HEART RATE TRAINING ZONE

SUBTRACT YOUR AGE FROM 200
(this will give you the maximum heart rate or upper limit of your training zone)

NEXT SUBTRACT 20 FROM THIS AMOUNT
(this will give you the middle of your training zone)

NOW SUBTRACT ANOTHER 20 FROM THIS AMOUNT (this will give you the minimum heart rate or lower limit of your training zone)

EXAMPLE
200–age (30 years)=170

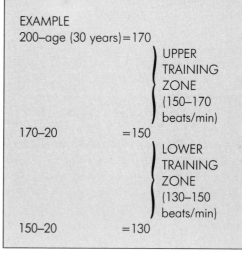

UPPER TRAINING ZONE (150–170 beats/min)

170–20　　　=150

LOWER TRAINING ZONE (130–150 beats/min)

150–20　　　=130

BUILD-UP AEROBICS

This exercise sequence gives you an idea of the sort of exercises which will improve your aerobic fitness. The exercises gradually grow in intensity by the inclusion of larger arm or leg movements as the sequence is repeated. It includes a number of variations in walking-type movements. Be sure to watch your posture as you move. There is usually a lead in to most music which gives you a chance to check your posture and stance before the real music for the exercise starts.

Starting Position

Stand with feet apart, knees soft, pelvis tucked under and tummy and pelvic floor muscles pulled in. Have your weight on both feet and your hands on hips.

Exercise 1

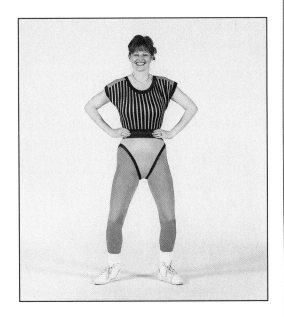

Knee bends × 2 slow.
Knee bends × 4 fast.

Exercise 2

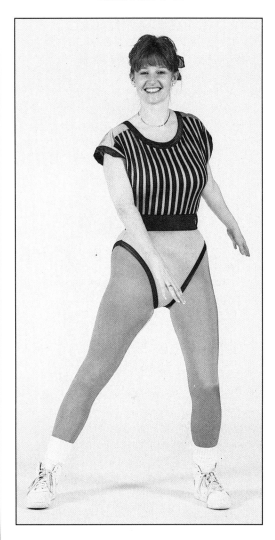

Lean your weight towards the left as you bend and lunge to the left, reaching down to the left knee with your right hand. Repeat to the right side. Do this 8 times, moving smothly and rhythmically from side to side. Repeat the exercise, this time with the opposite arm reaching out in front of you at shoulder height instead of down to your opposite knee. Do this 8 times, moving smoothly and rhythmically from side to side.

Exercise 3

Repeat exercise 1.

Exercise 4

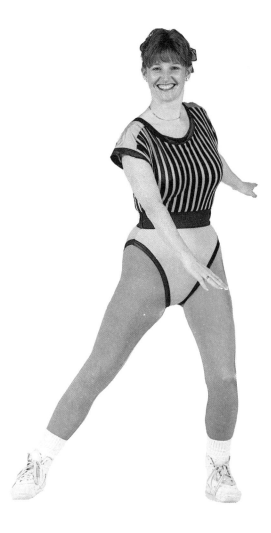

Transfer your weight from one foot to another as you stretch up and straighten first the right knee and then the left, bending both knees in the middle in between. Repeat with opposite arm reaching to opposite knee × 8. Repeat with opposite arm reaching out in front × 8.

Exercise 5

Repeat exercise 1.

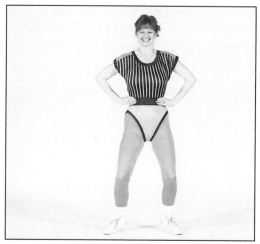

Knee bends × 2 slow.
Knee bends × 4 fast.

Exercise 6

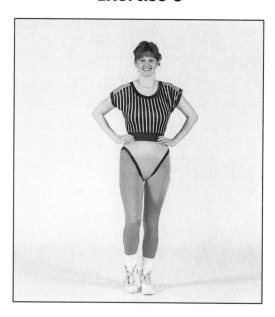

1 Step from side to side, tapping one foot beside the other (step, tap and step, tap). Do this 4 times. Hands on hips.

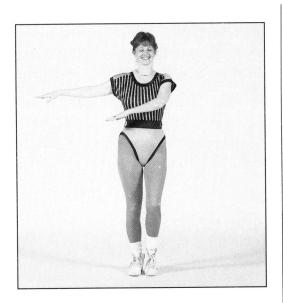

2 Repeat with both arms swinging from side to side 4 times. Repeat walking forwards i.e. with each step, step forwards and then tap. Do this 4 times. Walk backwards 1, 2, 3, 4.

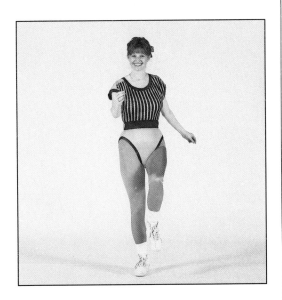

3 Mark time on the spot. Do this for 8 counts. Repeat walking sequence 4 times.

Exercise 7

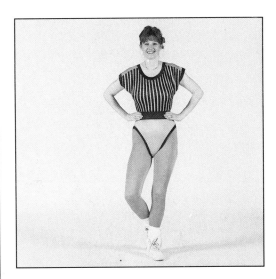

Step from side to side, tapping the toes of one foot behind the heel of the other. Hands on hips. Do this 8 times.

Exercise 8

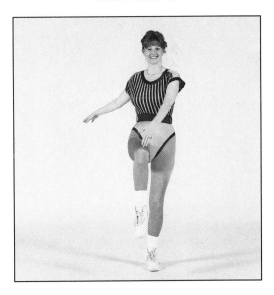

Lift alternate knees up in front of you to touch opposite hand on knee. Do this 8 times

Exercise 9

Step from side to side, lifting one foot behind off the ground to touch the heel with your opposite hand. Do this 8 times.

Exercise 10

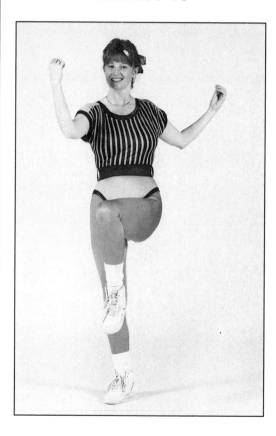

Repeat exercise 8 with elbow touching opposite knee. Do this 8 times.

Exercise 11

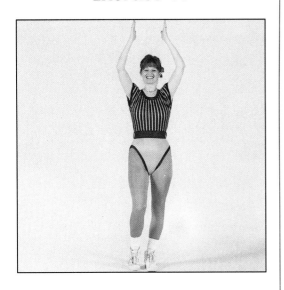

1 Walk forwards for 4 steps, clapping hands together above your head on the last step.

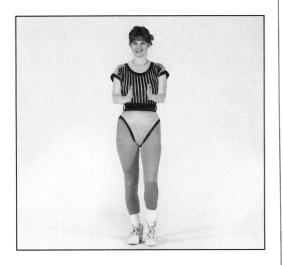

2 Walk backwards for 4 steps, clapping your hands together at waist height or below your knees on the last step. Repeat again. Now repeat 4 more times, each time walking to a different corner of the room to bring you round in a full circle back to the centre. Walk forwards and backwards twice more.

Exercising Time

When you first begin to do any aerobic-type exercise, you should begin slowly and build up gradually. You should aim to be working in your lower training zone for about 10–15 minutes, but at first you will probably only manage 2 or 3 minutes. You do not need to be working flat out at a high intensity throughout the whole 10 minutes. It is possible to stay within your training zone even though the intensity of the exercise varies, provided the intensity is enough to get you into your training zone in the first place.

Gradually increase the time you spend on the aerobic section. If your pulse rate shoots up into your upper training zone when you first start and you have only exercised for a few minutes, you may need to calm down the intensity a little, by keeping any movements small and the arms low. If you consistently work below your lower training zone, you will not be improving your cardiovascular fitness, although other aspects of fitness may improve. If you work at too high a level you could put unnecessary strain on your cardiovascular system and end up feeling worn out and not wanting to continue with your exercise programme.

As you get fitter, you can increase the time you are spending on the aerobic exercise section by incorporating the harder aerobic exercises. Always start at a low intensity and gradually build up to the harder exercises, then wind down slowly through the less intense exercises.

When you can comfortably manage to do 10 minutes in your lower training zone, you can then move into your upper training zone by increasing the length of time or the intensity of the exercises. You may then feel ready to move onto some classes or other form of activity. As you get fitter, you should be able to manage about 15–20 minutes of aerobic exercise quite easily.

HARD AEROBICS

In this section you need to work at a slightly faster rate or with larger movements, so that you are working harder than in the previous exercise sequence. Include some of these exercises as you get fitter.

The starting position for exercises 1–7 is standing with your feet together and your arms down by your side.

Exercise 1

March on the spot, raising both arms in front of you to a position above your head, to a count of 4 beats. March on the spot, bringing both hands down to the starting position by your side, shaking them out as you do so to a count of 4 beats. Repeat the sequence 4 times.

Exercise 2

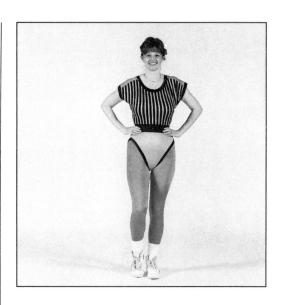

2 Repeat the whole stepping sequence twice to each side.

Exercise 3

Repeat exercise 1.

Exercise 4

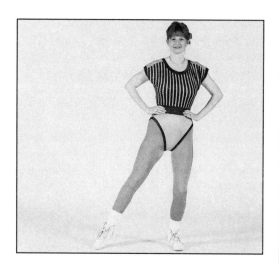

1 Step from side to side with a tap. Step to the right and tap with the left, step to the left and tap with the right. Do this 4 times. Then step to the right, bring the feet together, step to the right again and tap (step, together, step, tap). Hands on hips.

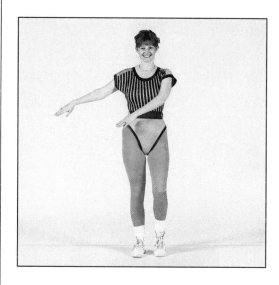

1 Repeat exercise 2, adding in the arms.

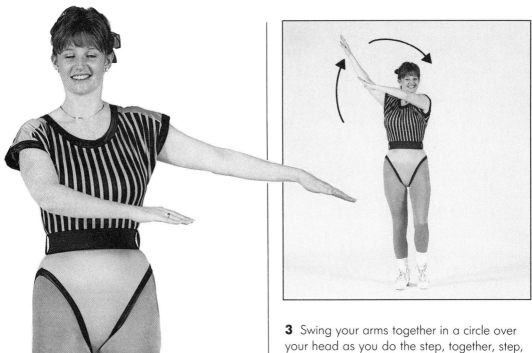

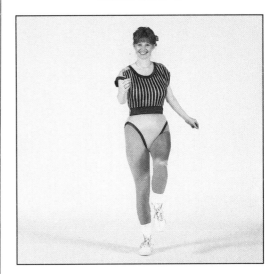

3 Swing your arms together in a circle over your head as you do the step, together, step, tap part of the sequence. Repeat to each side 4 times.

Exercise 5

March on the spot 4 times.

2 Swing your arms together from side to side as you step from side to side.

Exercise 6

Point your right leg straight out behind you, toe on the floor as you stretch your right arm straight out in front of you slightly above shoulder height. Alternate from side to side 8 times.

Exercise 7

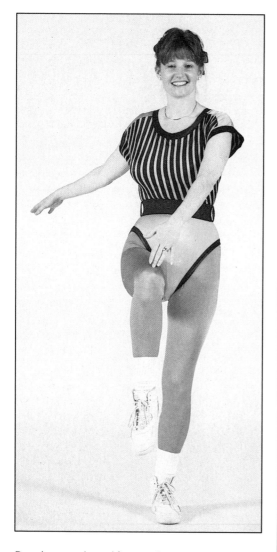

Do alternate knee lifts, touching opposite hand to the knee. Do this 8 times.

Exercise 8

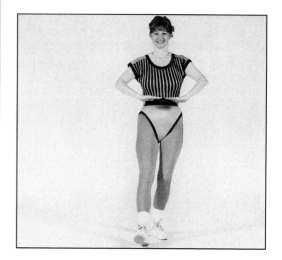

1 Stand with feet together and your hands at shoulder height with both elbows bent out to the side, palms facing the floor. Tap alternate heels in front of you at the same time pushing your arms down in front of you. Do this 8 times.

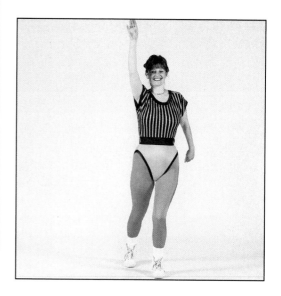

2 Point your right leg straight out behind you, toe on the floor as you push your right arm above your head and vice versa. Do this 8 times.

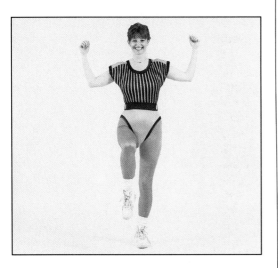

3 Do alternate knee lifts, stretching both arms above your head and, as you lift each knee, pull both arms down to shoulder height, closing the hands as if pulling down two ropes. Do this 8 times.

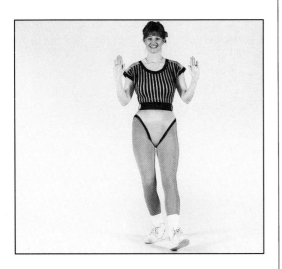

4 Tap alternate heels in front of you, pushing both arms out in front of you at shoulder height, palms facing away from your face. Do this 8 times.

Exercise 9

March on the spot 8 times.

Exercise 10

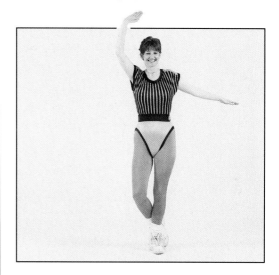

Stand with feet hip-width apart and your hands on your hips. Step from side to side, tapping one foot behind the other and swaying the arms from side to side at the same time. Do this 8 times.

WATCHPOINTS
● Remember to listen to your own body. If you feel very breathless or your heart is beating too fast, you will need to lower the intensity of the exercises as follows:
● lower the arms
● keep the knee bends shallow
● take smaller steps
● keep the knees low when doing knee lifts
● change from foot to foot keeping the toes on the ground, with gentle low arm swings instead of marching with vigorously swinging arms.

Exercise 11

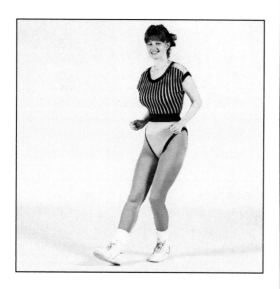

1 Step forward towards the right corner of the room on the right foot.

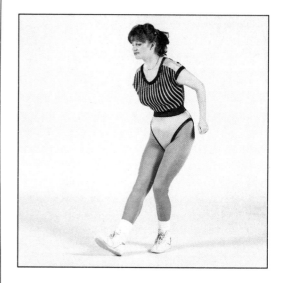

3 Step forwards again with the right and bring both feet together.

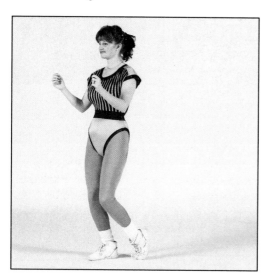

2 Bring the left foot to beside the right foot.

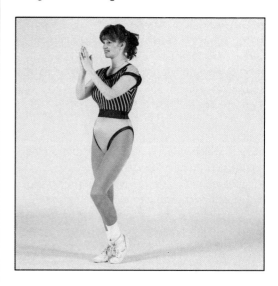

4 With each step, push forwards and back with your arms by your side bent at the elbows, clapping together in front as you bring the feet together (step together, step and clap). Repeat the sequence to the opposite corner. Do this twice.

MUSCULAR STRENGTH AND ENDURANCE SECTION (MSE)

There are many hundreds of muscles in your body responsible for posture and day-to-day activities. If muscles are not used they tend to become flabby and weak and a certain amount of wasting occurs. IF YOU DON'T USE IT YOU LOSE IT. On the first skylab missions, astronauts returned from space with very much reduced muscle volume through lack of use and are now given special resisted exercises to perform in space to reduce that muscle loss. This does not mean that you have to spend hours each day building up huge muscles. By doing just a few specific exercises you can influence most of the main important muscle groups. The effects of this type of exercise are as follows:

- Improvement in the strength of the muscles and the joints they help to support.
- Improvement in the condition of ligaments and tendons.
- Improvement in body shape as flabby muscles become firmer.
- As muscle balance returns, improvement in posture which in turn lessens the strain on the nerves and discs in the spine.
- Improvement in the ability to keep going for longer and with less fatigue.

To get the maximum benefit from this type of exercise it is necessary to understand some important principles about exercises and the way in which muscles work.

HOW MUSCLES WORK

Muscles usually work in opposing pairs to cause movement at the joints. A muscle on one side of the joint (known as the prime mover) contracts and the opposing muscle on the other side of the joint (the antagonist) has to relax to allow the movement to take place. At the same time, other muscles (the fixators) will be working to stabilise the working muscle's attachments to help it work more efficiently and prevent any unnecessary movement. For example, in bending the elbow, the biceps muscle at the front of the upper arm is the prime mover while the triceps muscle at the back of the upper arm is the antagonist and the shoulder girdle muscles are the fixators.

One particular type of contraction is called a concentric contraction. In the example given above, it involves the biceps muscle fibres shortening. When movement takes place in the opposite direction to return the joint to its original position, for example straightening the elbow, you would expect the triceps to be the prime mover but, because of the effects of gravity, this is not always the case. Straightening your elbow in the way described above actually still uses the biceps muscle. It is gravity which allows the arm to return to its normal position controlled by the biceps muscle in what is called an eccentric contraction with the fibres gradually lengthening to control the movement. This is one reason why as we get older the muscles at the back of the upper arms tend to get flabby. In normal everyday use they get little or no exercise. To prevent this tendency we have to do specific exercises which work these muscles against gravity or use some other resistance like body weight. For example, when doing curl-ups your abdominal muscles are working concentrically, when doing curl-downs they work eccentrically.

Knowing about these different kinds of contractions will help you to understand why following the instructions and getting into the right positions to perform the exercises is vital to ensure you work the correct muscles.

The contractions already mentioned are known as isotonic or dynamic contractions in which actual movement occurs. They are the best type of contractions to use in an exercise programme, although inevitably some muscles will be working statically at the same time. Static or isometric contraction occurs in muscles when you hold a limb in any one position for a length of time. Your biceps muscle would be in a static contraction if you held a shopping bag in your hand with your elbow bent in one position. No movement of limbs or joints occurs. The disadvantages of this type of contraction are:

• Muscle strength only improves in a very small, limited range of the muscles total range of capable movement.

• There is a tendency for blood pressure to rise when static contractions are performed and they should therefore be avoided by anyone with high blood pressure.

• Muscle fatigue and strains are more likely to occur with this type of exercise.

PRINCIPLES OF TRAINING

To improve the strength of a muscle you have to put a greater demand on it than you would do in normal day-to-day activities. You can achieve this increased loading on the muscles by increasing the frequency, intensity or duration of the exercise.

Frequency: Exercising 3 or 4 times a week is sufficient to show an improvement in muscle tone. The less fit you are the sooner you will begin to see some improvement. You can speed up progress by exercising more frequently but be careful to avoid overdoing it, especially in the early days.

Intensity: How hard you should exercise depends to a large extent on your level of fitness and should be determined by how you feel, although suggestions are made in the book about the number of repetitions. You

should always build up the intensity gradually and work to a level where you can feel some effects in the muscles, but stop before real fatigue sets in.

Intensity can be controlled by the number of repetitions of any given exercise, shortening the length of time you rest between repeated sets of the same exercise or by increasing the difficulty of the specific movement by adding weight or resistance. For example, 8 curl-ups with your hands sliding up your knees does not work your abdominal muscles as hard as 8 curl-ups with your hands behind your ears. This is because by raising the arms to the head you have altered the centre of gravity and increased the amount of body weight of the upper trunk to be lifted off the floor by the abdominals.

When you can perform 16–20 repetitions of the easier level comfortably you are ready to move on to the next level of diffculty.

Another way to increase intensity would be to do 2 or 3 sets of 8 exercises, interspersing each set with a different exercise for another muscle group or a very brief rest period. A low number of repetitions at a relatively high level of resistance will tend to improve muscle strength, while exercises of a relatively low level of resistance with a high number of repetitions will tend to improve muscle endurance.

Duration relates to the length of any exercise session. As you progress and get stronger, and as your baby grows, you will probably be able to spend longer doing your exercises. Initially it is important to concentrate on the main muscle groups affected by your pregnancy, mainly the pelvic floor and abdominal muscles. A total of 45 minutes is about the maximum you should need for the complete workout programme. If you can't find the time each day, it is possible to alternate. On one day you could concentrate on the strength section, the next day on the aerobic section but make sure you always include the warm-up, stretch and cool-down exercises each time. This would then cut down the time needed to about 15–20 minutes.

Guidelines

All the exercises in this Muscular Strength and Endurance (M.S.E) Section should be performed rhythmically and through as full a range of movement as possible, at a comfortable speed. Breathing should be even throughout the exercise.

Exercises for different muscle groups should be alternated so as to prevent undue fatigue in any one group of muscles.

You will only see results according to the particular exercises you have done. A well-balanced exercise programme includes all three fitness S's (Suppleness, Strength and Stamina).

Unfortunately you can't store fitness for the future and what you don't use, you lose. As we get older, we have a frequency to become less active and many of the changes that occur with ageing are thought to be due to this lack of activity, rather than any specific changes that occur with ageing. In normal everyday activity we very rarely move our joints through their full range of movement and over the years this range of movement gradually gets smaller.

The difficulty that elderly people often experience with dressing or combing their hair is probably due to the fact that they have hardly ever raised their arms fully above their head and so the shoulder joints have become stiff and the shoulder muscles weakened. Weak muscles cannot move stiff joints very effectively and, consequently, the range of movement gradually diminishes.

Only regular exercise will ensure that you maintain full joint movement and muscle strength so IF YOU WANT TO BE ABLE TO DO SOMETHING TOMORROW, DO IT TODAY.

In this muscular strength and endurance section you will see that some of the exercises have different levels of difficulty. This is to enable you to progress through your own exercise programme as you become fitter.

Start with 6–8 repetitions and gradually build up to about 15–20. When you can perform 15–20 repetitions of an exercise comfortably, you are probably ready to move on to the next stage of difficulty. If you then find you can't perform 6 full repetitions of the harder stage it may mean that this stage is too hard for you. Go back to the previous stage for a bit longer. When you can manage 6 of the harder stage you can try combining the 2 stages for a while, doing as many as you can of the harder stage without strain while still doing some at the easier level. Once you can do 8–10 of the harder level, it is best to concentrate on that stage alone and not bother with the easier stage.

If your muscles shake or you feel very tired, so that the quality of movement is getting worse with each repetition, this is a sign that you have worked that muscle hard enough. Stop that particular exercise and try a different exercise for another muscle group. If the shaking occurs after only a few repetitions, the level is too hard. Go back to previous stage.

Before starting the abdominal exercises in this section (see page 70), do the Rec Check described on page 15 to make sure that any separation in your rectus abdominus muscles has narrowed up to about two finger widths or less. DO NOT ATTEMPT THE STRONGER CURL-UPS OR DIAGONAL CURL-UPS UNTIL IT HAS DONE SO.

Watch your tummy for signs of bulging. Keep the muscles firmly contracted to avoid this. If the separation is still wide, continue to do the basic curl-up with your hands across your abdomen as shown on page 26, trying to gradually increase the number of repetitions you do each time and trying to do the exercises more often.

ABDOMINAL MUSCLE EXERCISES

Aim: To strengthen the rectus abdominus muscles. The action of this muscle is to bend the head and shoulders forwards on the trunk to approximately 45 degrees. You should not aim to get yourself all the way up into a sitting position from lying on your back. Keeping your waist on the ground as you raise your head and shoulders will ensure that you work only the abdominal muscles. Never anchor your feet under furniture as this is liable to cause back strain because you bring into play the strong hip flexor muscles which are attached to the lower spine. Never do straight leg sit-ups, as in this position it is impossible to keep the small of the back safely pressed into the floor.

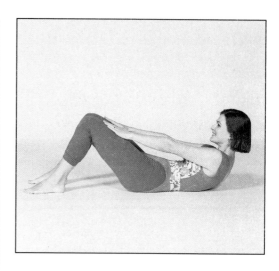

2 Tuck your chin in and look at your knees. Slowly uncurl back to the starting position. If you feel any strain in your neck you can help to support your head with one hand, but be careful not to pull on your neck as you curl up. Repeat 6–8 times, progressing to 16 before moving to next level.

Curl-ups: Level 1

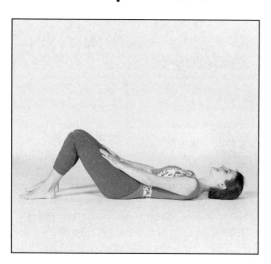

1 Lie on your back with your knees bent, and your feet flat on the floor. Breathe in and as you breathe out, pull in your abdominal muscles, pressing the small of your back flat into the floor and slide both hands up your thighs towards your knees.

Curl-ups: Level 2

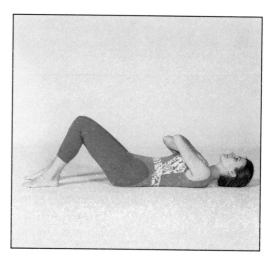

1 As curl-ups: level 1 except that your hands should be crossed over your chest instead of resting on your thighs.

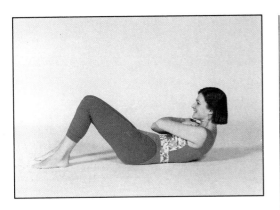

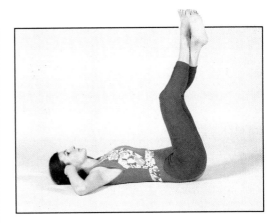

2 Tuck your chin in and look at your knees as before. Repeat 6–8 times, progressing to 16 repetitions before moving onto the next level.

Curl-ups: Level 3

Lie on your back with both knees bent, hands beside your ears. Keeping your abdominal muscles firmly contracted and your back flat on the floor throughout the exercise, bend your right knee, bringing it in towards your chest and at the same time lifting your head and shoulders off the floor towards your knee. Repeat 6–8 times before changing legs and repeating.

Curl-ups: Level 4

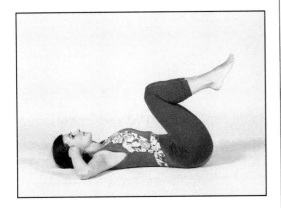

1 Lie on your back, hands beside your ears. Bend both knees up towards your chest.

2 Cross your ankles and straighten your legs up towards the ceiling until they are directly above your hips with slightly bent knees.

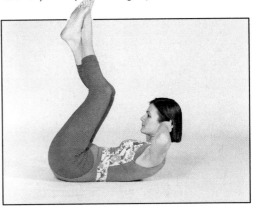

3 Breathe in and as you breathe out, pull in your abdominal muscles and curl your head and shoulders up off the floor towards your knees. Make sure that your knees remain directly over your hips and that your back is flat on the floor. Repeat 6–8 times, progressing to 16 repetitions. At the end of the exercise, hug both knees in to your chest for a few seconds and relax with your back pressed flat against the floor, then slowly lower your feet back onto the floor into a bent knees position.

• • • • •

Alternative Level 4 with Baby

1 Lie on your back with your knees bent up towards your chest and knees directly over your hips. Hold your baby in position along your shins.

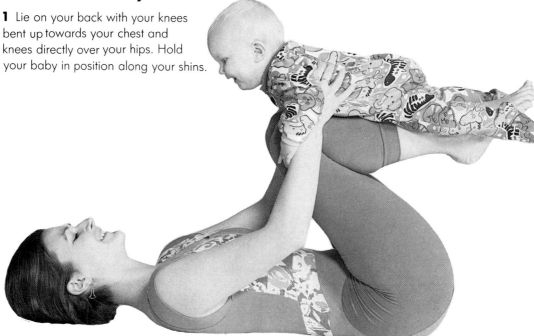

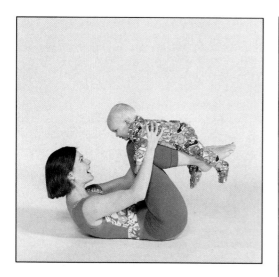

2 Raise your head and shoulders off the floor as you come up straight to kiss your baby on the nose or forehead. Keep your tummy muscles pulled in as you do this.

....

WATCHPOINTS

● Take care not to twist getting into this position. Sit with your knees bent, holding your baby on your knees. Curl down into a lying position then bend your knees onto your chest and lift the baby onto your shins as you do so.

....

Diagonal Curl-ups

Aim: To strengthen the oblique abdominal muscles. The main action of these muscles is to flex the trunk diagonally, for example bending one shoulder down and across towards the opposite hip. When all the abdominal muscles on one side work together they bend the trunk sideways.

Diagonal Curl-ups: Level 1

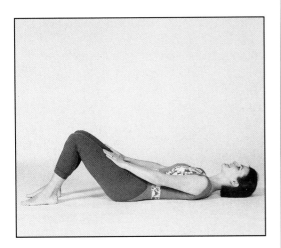

1 Lie on your back with your knees bent, feet flat on the floor. Breathe in and as you breathe out pull in your abdominal muscles and press your back flat against the floor.

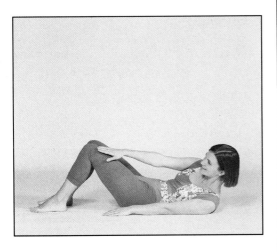

2 Tuck your chin in and slide your right hand up and across your left thigh as far as the outside of your left knee. Return to the starting position and repeat on the other side. Do 6–8 times on each side, progressing to 16 repetitions before moving on to the next stage.

Diagonal Curl-ups: Level 2

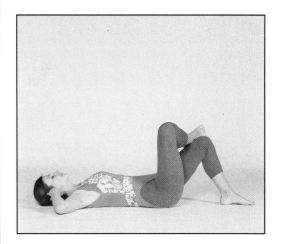

1 Lie on your back with your knees bent, place your right ankle across your left knee. Keep the right knee pressed away from your body. Place both hands beside your ears.

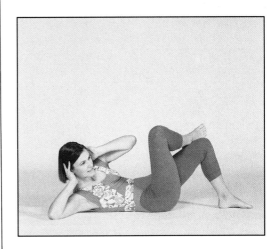

2 Breathe in and as you breathe out, pull in your abdominal muscles and raise your head and shoulders off the floor bringing your left elbow up and across in the direction of your right knee. Keep your right elbow on the floor. Return to the start position and repeat 6–8 times before changing to the other side. Progress to 16 repetitions before moving on.

Diagonal Curl-ups: Level 3

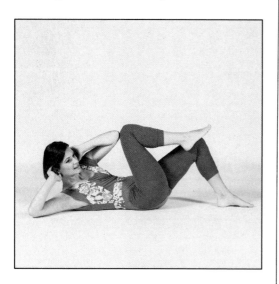

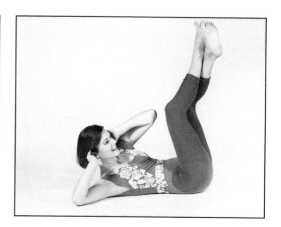

Lie on your back with both knees bent, hands beside your ears and chin tucked in. Keep your abdominal muscles firmly contracted and your back flat on the floor throughout the exercise. Bend your right knee, bringing it in towards your chest and at the same time lifting your head and shoulders off the floor to bring your left elbow across towards your right knee. Repeat 6–8 times before changing legs.

Breathe in and as you breathe out, pull in your abdominal muscles and lift your head and shoulders off the floor, bringing your left elbow to your right knee and then lowering it back to the floor before repeating to the opposite side. Repeat 6–8 times each side. Bend both knees onto your chest and slowly lower your feet to the floor keeping both knees bent.

Alternative Level 4 Diagonal Curl-ups with Baby

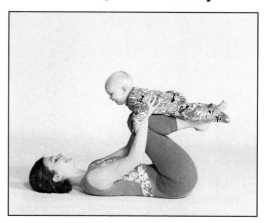

Diagonal Curl-ups: Level 4

Lie on your back, bend both knees up towards your chest. Cross your ankles and straighten your legs up towards the ceiling until they are directly above your hips with knees slightly bent and separated. Place both hands behind your ears and keep your chin tucked in.

1 Lie on your back with your knees bent up towards your chest and knees directly over your hips. Hold your baby in position on her tummy along your shins.

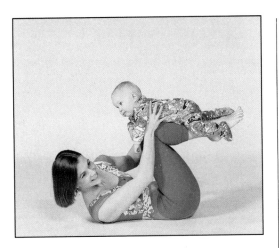

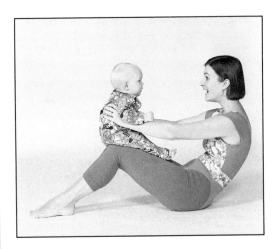

2 Raise your head and shoulders off the floor as you come up diagonally to alternately kiss your baby's ear first on one side and then on the other.

Curl-down

This exercise can be done as an alternative to curl-ups.

2 Breathe in and as you breathe out, keep your abdominal muscles firmly contracted, relax and round your back and curl-down vertebra by vertebra halfway towards a lying position, until you feel the abdominal muscles working quite hard, but not feeling too much strain. Return to the starting position. Repeat 6–8 times.

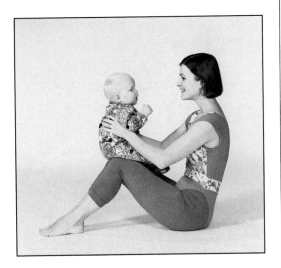

1 Sit up straight with your knees bent, feet flat on the floor and with your baby sitting on your knees facing you, or on your tummy with her back resting against your thighs.

WATCHPOINTS FOR ALL ABDOMINAL EXERCISES
● Pull in the abdominal muscles before starting any exercise to ensure a safe, flat back. Don't allow the muscles to bulge or dome.
● Breathe out on the effort.
● Keep hands beside ears and not pulling on neck.

UPPER BODY EXERCISES

Aim: To strengthen the muscles of the upper chest and arms which are mainly responsible for lifting and carrying. As your baby gets older and heavier, you will need stronger muscles to carry her around. The triceps muscles at the back of the upper arms, which tend to get flabby through lack of use, are strengthened when you do these exercises.

Wall Press-ups: Level 1

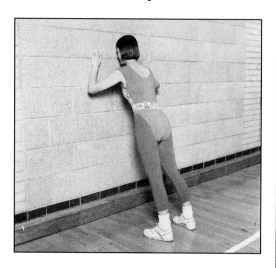

Stand with your feet hip-width apart and your body about an arm's length away from the wall. Place both your hands flat on the wall at shoulder height. Breathing evenly throughout, bend your elbows and lower your body so that your chin almost touches the wall between your hands. Squeeze your buttocks together and pull in your abdominal muscles and let your heels come off the floor slightly, to ensure that you keep your body in a straight line. Don't bend forwards at the waist or hollow your back. Push yourself back to the starting position, lowering the heels. Repeat 6–8 times and progress up to 16 repetitions before moving on to the next level.

Table Press-ups: Level 2

Stand with your feet hip-width apart and far enough away from a firm and immovable table so that when you place your hands on the edge of the table, shoulder-width apart, your body leans towards the table at an angle of about 45 degrees. Keeping your buttocks and abdominal muscles contracted and your back flat, bend at the elbows and lower yourself down towards the table so that your chest almost touches the table between your hands. Push yourself back into the starting position. Repeat 6–8 times and progress up to 16 repetitions before moving on to the next level.

Alternate Level-2: Push-ups with the Baby

If you have your baby lying on a table or work top the correct height for nappy changing, you could incorporate your table press-ups.

....

WATCHPOINTS
- If the muscles shake or you are unable to do at least 6 repetitions easily it means you have chosen too hard a level. Go back to the previous level.
- Keep your shoulders relaxed away from your ears.
- Keep your bottom tucked under to make sure your body stays in a straight line.
- Breathe evenly throughout the exercise. (You may find it easier to breathe out on the effort i.e. as you push up.)

....

Box Press-ups: Level 3

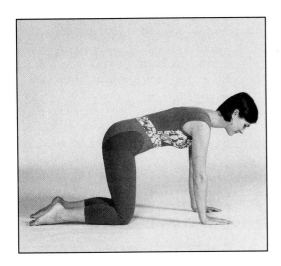

1 Kneel on the floor with your hands directly under your shoulders and your knees directly under your hips. Pull in your abdominal muscles and keep your back flat throughout the exercise.

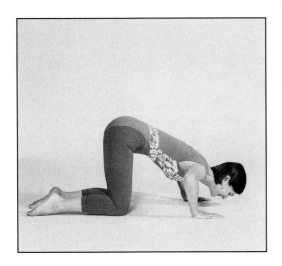

2 Bend your elbows and lower your body towards the floor. Push yourself back up into the starting position. Repeat 6–8 times and progress up to 16 repetitions before moving on to the next level.

Modified Floor Press-ups: Level 4

Lie face down on the floor, cross your feet at the ankles and bend your knees. Place your hands on the floor directly underneath your shoulders. Push yourself up onto the soft part of the thigh just above your knees. Your body should be in a straight line from knees to shoulders. Pull in your abdominal muscles and keep your back flat throughout the exercise by squeezing your buttocks together.

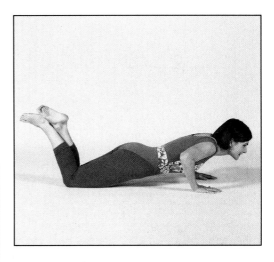

Bend your elbows and lower your body towards the floor. Repeat 6–8 times and progress up to 16 repetitions. If you can't do 6 of this last stage well, without resting your body on the floor in between each press-up, it is too hard for you.

....

WATCHPOINTS
● With the press-ups, it is important that all the movement occurs at the elbows and not at the waist. There should be no discomfort in your elbow or shoulder joints.

....

Alternative to Press-ups
Tricep Dips: Level 1

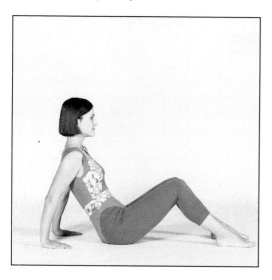

1 Sit with your knees bent, feet flat on the floor and your hands placed behind you with your fingers facing forwards.

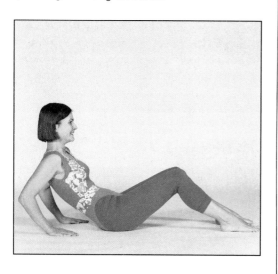

2 Bend your elbows and lower yourself towards the floor, then push up back to the starting position. Don't lock the elbows into a straight position. Repeat 6–8 times and progress up to 15 repetitions.

Tricep Dips: Level 2

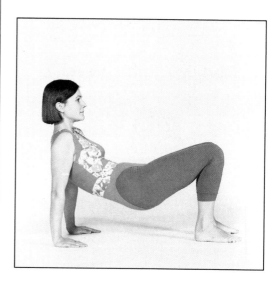

1 Sit as for triceps dips: level 1, take the weight on your hands and raise your buttocks a few inches off the floor.

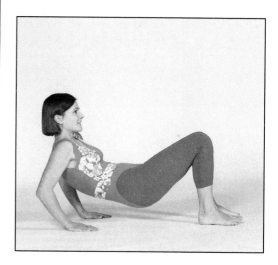

2 Now bend and straighten the elbows to work the triceps more strongly.

• • • • • •

LEG EXERCISES

Aim: To strengthen the outer hip and main thigh muscles.

Abductor Lifts: Level 1

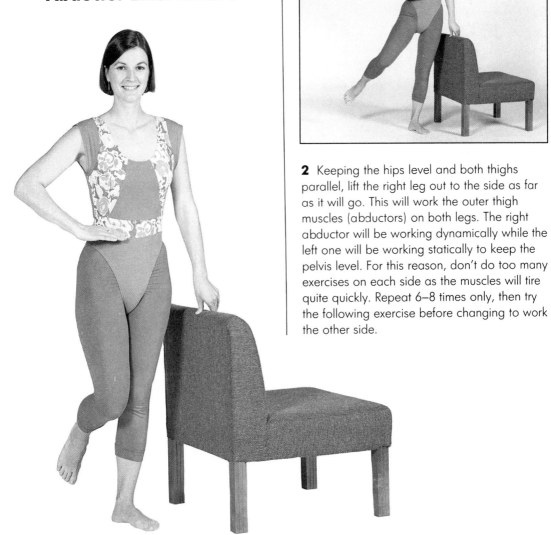

2 Keeping the hips level and both thighs parallel, lift the right leg out to the side as far as it will go. This will work the outer thigh muscles (abductors) on both legs. The right abductor will be working dynamically while the left one will be working statically to keep the pelvis level. For this reason, don't do too many exercises on each side as the muscles will tire quite quickly. Repeat 6–8 times only, then try the following exercise before changing to work the other side.

1 Stand with your feet together, holding onto a chair with your left hand. Bend the right leg at the knee with the foot out behind you.

Quadriceps Squats

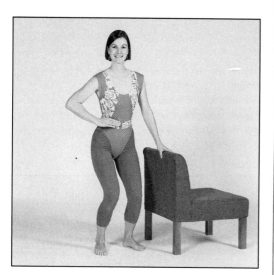

Stand beside the chair holding on to it with your left hand and with your feet about 60 cm (2 feet) apart. Keeping your back straight, bend both knees as if you were about to sit down on a chair. Do not go all the way down. This works the large muscles on the front of the thighs (quadriceps). Return to the upright position. Repeat 6–8 times, then turn to face the other way and repeat this and the previous exercise on the other side.

....

WATCHPOINTS
- Keep the body upright as you bend the knees.
- Full knee bends tend to cause strain on the knee joints. Only bend as far as you would need if you were going to sit on a chair.
- Keep the knees directly over your toes. Don't allow the knees to roll inwards towards each other as this can strain the knees.
- Keep your heels on the ground as this will help you to avoid deep knee bends.

....

Hamstring Curls: Level 1

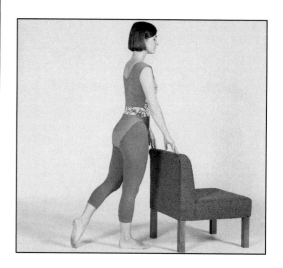

1 Stand with your feet hip-width apart, facing the chair with hands resting on it. Keeping your hips facing forwards and level, and with weight on your hands and right leg, point left toe onto floor behind you, as far as it will go.

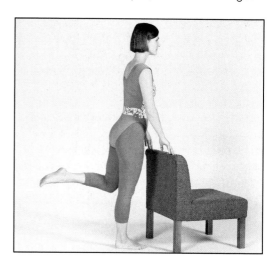

2 Keeping the left thigh at that angle, bend the knee and then straighten it again. This should work your gluteal (buttock) muscles and hamstring muscles at back of left thigh. Repeat 6–8 times; change to the other leg.

Abductor Lifts: Level 2

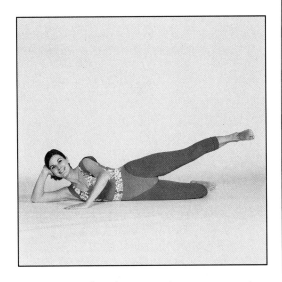

Lie on your right side propped up on your right elbow with both hips facing forwards and the upper hip directly above the lower one. Keep your body in a straight line and your abdominal muscles pulled in. Bend the right knee and place your left hand in front of you for stability. Lift the left leg as far as it will go and then lower. This exercise will work the hip and outer thigh muscles of the left leg strongly. Keep your upper hip pushed well forwards or you will find you can lift the leg really high but you will be working the wrong muscles. Repeat 6–8 times, progressing to 16 repetitions in 2 sets of 8 with a short rest in between if necessary, before changing to lie on the left side and work the right leg. You can vary the exercise by doing one set with your foot bent up at the ankle and one set with your toes pointed.

....

WATCHPOINT FOR GLUTEALS AND HAMSTRINGS SQUEEZES

- Each time you lift remember to contract those abdominal muscles and press the back onto the floor.

....

Gluteals and Hamstrings Squeeze: Level 1

The gluteals and hamstrings exercises work the muscles at the back of the thigh and buttocks. The variation can include inner thighs and pelvic floor muscles as well.

Lie on your back with your knees bent and feet flat on the floor and slightly apart. Breathe in and as you breathe out, pull in your abdominal muscles to keep your back flat on the floor. Squeeze your buttocks together and release. Repeat 6–8 times, progressing to 16.

Gluteals and Hamstrings Squeeze: Level 2

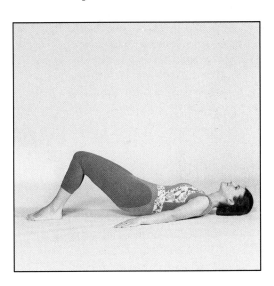

Lie on your back with your knees bent and feet flat on the floor and slightly apart. Breathe in and as you breathe out, pull in your abdominal muscles to keep your back flat on the floor. Squeeze your buttocks together and lift them a few inches off the floor. Release and return to the floor. Repeat 6–8 times, progressing to 16 repetitions.

• • • • • •

Buttock and Adductor Squeeze Variation

As the previous exercise, but as you squeeze and lift, press your thighs together working the inner thigh muscles (adductors), relaxing the thighs apart as you lower the buttocks. Repeat 6–8 times, eventually progressing to 16 repetitions. Once you are confident that you know how to contract your pelvic floor muscles independently, you can include them in this exercise as follows. Squeeze and lift the buttocks, pressing the inner thighs together. Hold while you pull up your pelvic floor as well and then release back to the floor.

Adductor Lifts: Level 2

Lie flat on your right side with your head resting on your right hand. Bend your left knee and cross the left leg over in front of the right leg, placing the left lower leg on the floor. Keeping the right leg straight and the right foot flexed at the ankle with the foot turned slightly up towards the ceiling, lift the right leg up a few inches off the floor and lower. Rhythmically repeat the lift and lower 6–8 times, progressing to 16 repetitions before changing to the other side.

WATCHPOINTS
- Keep the knee straight as you lift the whole leg from the floor.
- Use a mat or towel if you find lying your hip bone is uncomfortable.
- Keeping the inner border of the foot turned towards the ceiling ensures that the adductor muscles are working properly.
- Place your left hand on the floor out in front of you to stabilise your position.

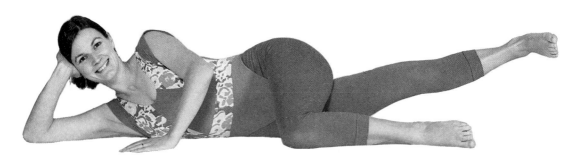

BACK EXERCISES

Aim: The erector spinae are muscles which run the full length of the back. They are important, in conjunction with the abdominal muscles, in maintaining good posture. It is important that the two opposing sets of muscles are balanced. Following pregnancy, it is likely that your erector spinae muscles are much stronger than your abdominal muscles. Although the abdominals require more intensive exercising, it is important to exercise the back muscles as well.

Cat Arch: Level 1

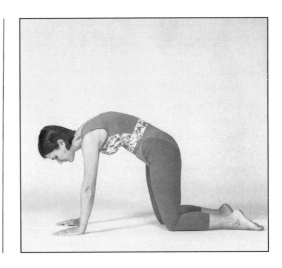

2 Breathe in and as you breathe out, pull in your abdominal muscles and drop your head onto your chest, rounding your back up towards the ceiling like an angry cat. Release and return to the starting position, lifting your head as you do so. Be careful not to let your back sag or dip too much. This exercise will work the abdominal muscles when you round the back, and the erector spinae muscles will contract as you raise your head. Repeat 6–8 times, progressing to 16 repetitions.

1 Kneel on all-fours with your hands directly under your shoulders and your knees, slightly apart, directly under your hips.

WATCHPOINTS
- Make sure you use your abdominal
  - Remember to breathe evenly throughout the exercise.
- Keep the movements slow and rhythmical.

Prone Kneeling Alternate Leg Lifts: Level 2

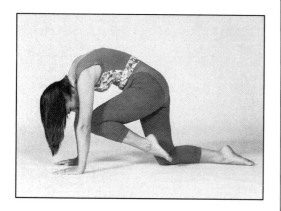

Kneel on all-fours with your hands directly under your shoulders and your knees, slightly apart, directly under your hips. Bend your head down onto your chest and bend the left knee towards the head, rounding your back as you do so. Lift the head level with your back and stretch the left leg straight out behind you (see below). Do this in a slow and controlled movement. Take care not to lift the back leg too high or let your back dip and arch as you straighten the leg out behind you. Repeat 6–8 times before changing legs. Progress to doing 2 sets of 8 on each leg, alternating rather than doing 16 on one leg.

Prone, Lying Alternate Leg Lifts, (for Lower Erector Spinae Muscles and Gluteal Muscles of the Buttocks): Level 3

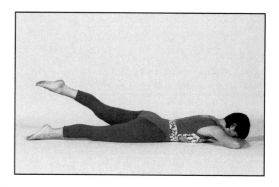

Lie face down on the floor, elbows bent and with your forehead resting on your hands. Lift your left leg straight up behind you. It will not lift very far and it is important to keep both hips flat on the floor and not to feel any strain or pain in the lower back. Repeat 6–8 times before changing to the other leg. Progress to 2 sets of 8 on each side rather than 16 all on the one side.

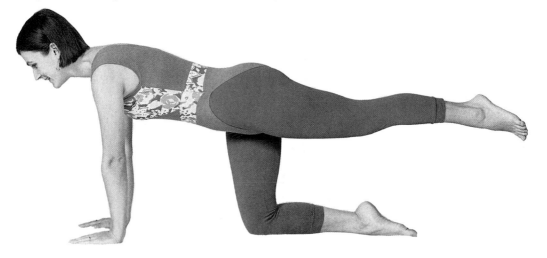

Prone Lying Head and Shoulder Lifts (for Upper Erector Spinae Muscles): Level 2

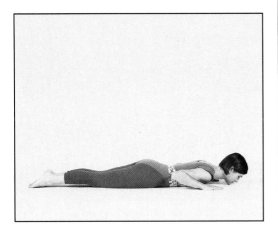

1 Lie face down with your hands resting under your shoulders.

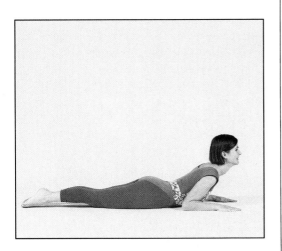

2 Press down on your hands and lift your head and shoulders no more than about 25 cm (10 inches) off the floor, keeping both hips flat on the floor. You shouldn't experience any pain or strain in the lower back. Repeat 6–8 times, progressing to 16 by doing 2 sets of 8 with a short rest in between.

Prone Lying Head and Shoulder Lifts (for Upper Erector Spinae Muscles): Level 3

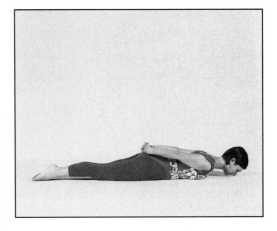

1 Lie face down with your forehead resting on the floor and hands clasped behind your back.

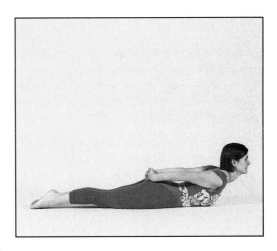

2 Breathe in and as you breathe out, lift your head and shoulders off the ground, pulling your hands down towards your feet.

• • • • • •

TYPICAL MSE WORKOUT

This exercise programme is designed for you to be able to work at your own level. You may find that you need to be exercising at level 1 for one group of muscles and level 3 for another. Below are some suggestions of how to put together a set of different MSE exercises, chosen for your own personal level of fitness from the exercises described on the previous pages. The number of repetitions suggested are the minimum. When you feel ready to progress, increase the number as suggested, before progressing to the next level of difficulty for that exercise.

Do the following exercise standing.

EXERCISE 1: Wall press-ups × 8 (see page 76)

EXERCISE 2: see Abductor lifts: Level 1 × 8 (for the right leg, page 79)

EXERCISE 3: Quadriceps squats × 4 (see page 80)

EXERCISE 4: Hamstring curls × 8 (for the right leg, see page 80)

EXERCISE 5: Repeat exercise 2 (for the left leg)

EXERCISE 6: Repeat exercise 3 × 4

EXERCISE 9: Repeat exercise 4 (for the left leg)

Get down onto floor in crook lying position (on your back with knees bent, feet flat on the floor) for the following exercises.

EXERCISE 10: Pelvic floor squeeze × 6 (see page 27)   ☆

EXERCISE 11: Abdominal curl-ups × 8 (see page 26)   ☆

EXERCISE 12: Gluteal squeezes × 8 (see page 81)

EXERCISE 13: Diagonal curl-ups × 8 (see page 73)   ☆

EXERCISE 14: Pelvic floor lift × 8 (see page 27)   ☆

Do the next exercise in a prone kneeling position (on all-fours).

EXERCISE 15: Cat arch × 8 (see page 83)   ☆

Return to the sitting position for the last exercise.

EXERCISE 16: Curl-downs × 8 (see page 75)   ☆

Well done! You have reached the end of the main exercise sections. Now enjoy a good stretch and relax into the cool-down.
   Lie on your back, hug both knees into your chest and rock gently from side to side for a few seconds. Now place your feet back on the floor and slide your legs out straight. Stretch out both arms above your head and enjoy a really good stretch.

STRETCH AND COOL-DOWN SECTION

These stretch exercises help your muscles relax before you do the final cool-down.

Hamstring Stretch

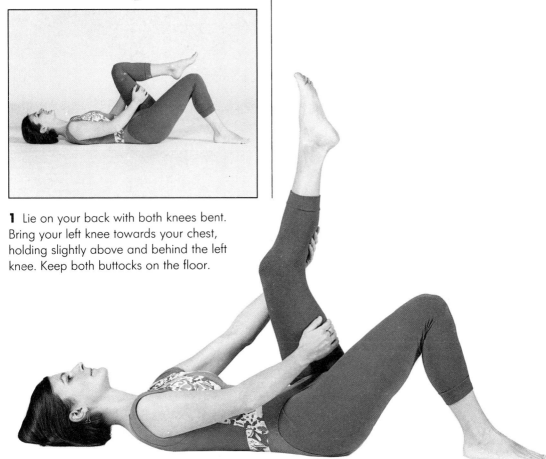

1 Lie on your back with both knees bent. Bring your left knee towards your chest, holding slightly above and behind the left knee. Keep both buttocks on the floor.

2 You can gradually straighten the left leg to increase the stretch, but it does not have to be completely straight. You should feel a stretch behind the left thigh. Make sure it is a gradual stretch and don't bounce. Hold for 6–8 seconds, then replace the foot on the floor and repeat on the other side.

Gluteal Stretch

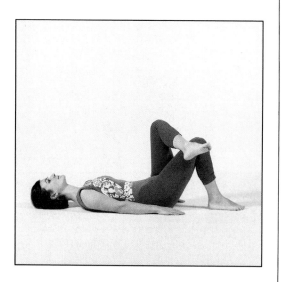

1 Lie on your back with both knees bent. Place your left ankle across the right knee.

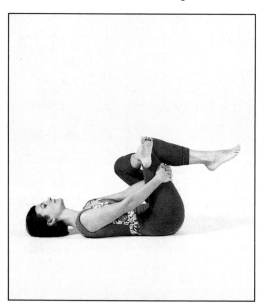

2 Place both hands behind your right thigh and lift the right leg towards your chest. You should feel a stretch across the left buttock. Hold for 6–8 seconds.

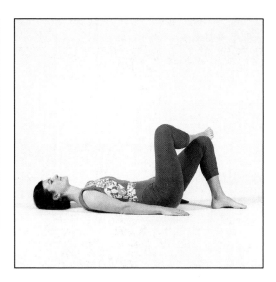

3 Repeat for the other leg. Replace both feet on the floor. Slowly roll onto your side.

Quadriceps Stretch

Lie on your left side, keep your legs straight and your knees together and bend the right leg.

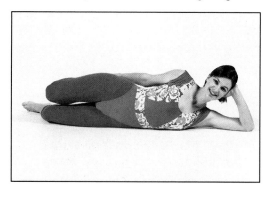

Clasp your right ankle with your right hand and gently ease the right thigh back behind the level of the left thigh. You should feel a stretch on the front of the right thigh. Keep your pelvis tucked forwards to avoid arching your back. Hold for a few seconds, then roll onto your left side and repeat with the left leg. Slowly push yourself up into a sitting position.

Adductor Stretch

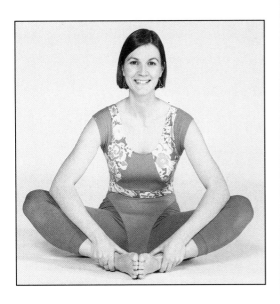

Sit with the soles of your feet touching each other and knees bent. Hold your ankles with your hands and, with your elbows resting on your knees gently lean forward and ease your thighs apart as far as they will go. You should feel the stretch in the inner thighs. Hold for 6–8 seconds, gradually easing them further as the muscles relax, but don't bounce.

....

WATCHPOINTS
● If the adductor stretch feels very uncomfortable, ease your feet a little further away from the body. Easing your feet nearer towards your body will increase the adductor stretch further.
● Keep your head up straight on the triceps stretch. Don't poke your chin forwards as you concentrate on the stretch.
● Always perform stretches slowly and smoothly. No bouncing.

....

Triceps Stretch

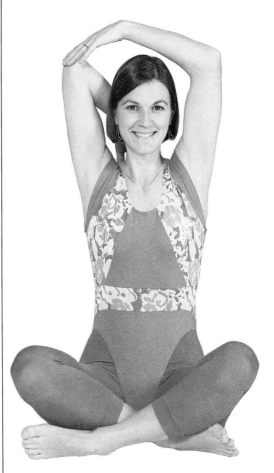

Sit with your ankles crossed, abdominal muscles pulled in and back straight. Stretch your right arm above your head, close to your ear. Bend your elbow and place your right hand down behind you. Take your left hand across and clasp the right elbow and gently ease it towards the left. You should feel a stretch in the back of the right upper arm. Hold for a few seconds and repeat on the other side.

● ● ● ● ● ●

HEAD AND NECK EXERCISES

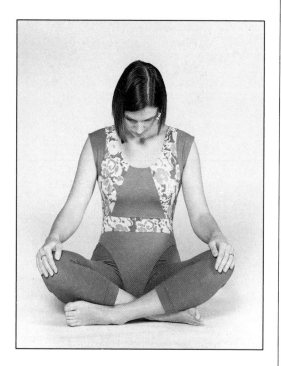

1 Sit with knees bent and your ankles crossed. Hands relaxed on your knees or thighs or on the floor beside you. Flex your head slowly forward onto your chest until you feel a slight stretch down back of neck.

....

WATCHPOINTS
• These exercises should always be done slowly.
• Work within your own range of movement. Do not force your head too far in any direction especially not backwards.
• Concentrate on relaxing the shoulders down away from the ears.

....

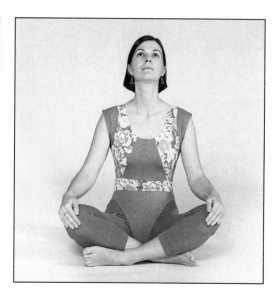

2 Return to the centre and then look carefully upwards. DO NOT THROW YOUR HEAD RIGHT BACK and look up at the ceiling above your head as this puts undue pressure on the discs in the cervical spine. Repeat a few times, ensuring that the movement is smooth.

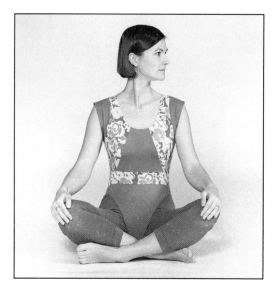

3 Turn your head to look over your left shoulder as far as is comfortable.

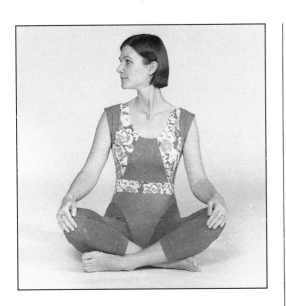

4 Repeat to the right. Repeat a few times with a smooth and gentle rhythm.

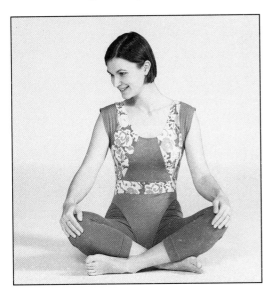

5 Then look left and swing the head gently down and across the chest in a half circle to look to the right. Repeat to the left, then a few times in each direction.

• • • • • •

Side Stretch

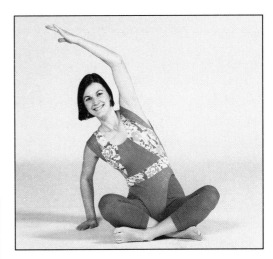

Still sitting, place your right hand on the floor beside you. Lean towards the right hand and stretch the left arm above your head. Keep the arm slightly in front of your head to avoid back arching. You should feel the stretch all down your left side. Hold for a few seconds and then repeat on the other side. Slowly come up to standing position as described on page 24.

Gastrocnemius Stretch

Stand facing and close to a wall and place the toes of your right foot in front of you against the wall, while resting your right heel on the floor. Keep the knee straight but avoiding locking it back too hard, then gently ease your weight over the right leg pressing your whole body nearer to the wall until you feel a stretch in the back of the right calf. Hold for a few seconds and then change legs and repeat with the left leg.

Move away from the wall and stand with feet hip width apart, knees soft and tummy tucked in for the final cool-down exercises.

• • • • • •

COOL-DOWN

Arm Circling

Aim: To slowly and rhythmically return the body to a non-exercising status.

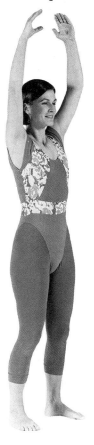

Stand tall with feet hip-width apart, knees soft, pelvis tucked under and shoulders back and down. Circle your arms forwards close to your ears and then over your head in a full circle, bending your knees as your arms come down past your thighs and straightening the knees as your arms go over your head. Take a deep breath in as you reach upwards. Repeat 4–6 times rhythmically.

Foot Circling

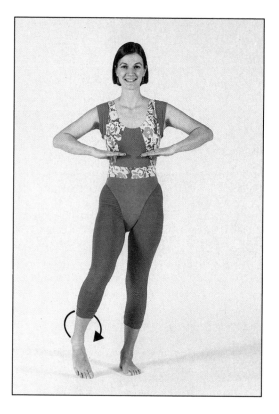

Stand on one foot and rest the toes of the other foot on the floor and circle your ankle a few times, keeping your toes in contact with the floor. Repeat in the other direction and then change feet.

....

WATCHPOINTS
• It is important after exercising to gradually return the body to the pre-exercise state and not stop suddenly. Large amounts of blood will be circulating through the muscles you have been using and suddenly stopping the exercises could lead to feeling faint.

....

Pelvic Tilting and Circling

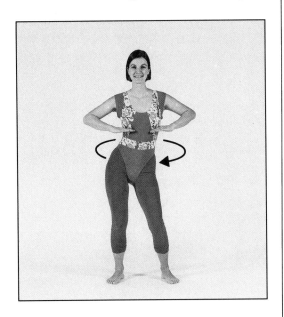

Stand as pelvic tilt and circles, page 46.

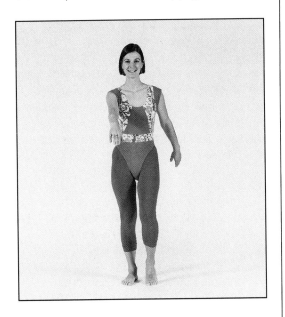

Mark time on the spot, always keeping the toes of one foot on the ground as you change from foot to foot.

AFTER THE EXERCISE SESSION

Finish your exercise programme with a couple of large arm circles, each with a deep breath in as you take the arms above your head.

Exercise releases the body's natural endorphins (pain relieving compounds) which can elevate your mood. At the end of the exercise session you should feel refreshed, relaxed and envigorated. If, on the other hand, you feel exhausted and unable to do anything else for the rest of the day, you have worked at a level which was too difficult for you and you need to modify your programme.

As you learn more about your body and the way it functions, you will gain more from your exercise sessions. If you find it hard to keep motivated, try to find an appropriate exercise class or other exercise activity, such as badminton or swimming, which you might enjoy and where you can meet other mothers.

The NCT has recently embarked on a training programme for postnatal exercise teachers. These classes also include group discussions on all sorts of topics of interest to new mothers and are proving to be very popular.

> 66 The PNEX classes were very good. Great fun and interesting. 99

Contact the NCT's Postnatal Committee to see if there is a postnatal exercise teacher near you. For further information see Useful Addresses at the end of the book.

Your changing role

It is hard to imagine beforehand how you will feel at the moment when you first lift your new-born baby into your arms and you suddenly realise you have become a mother. You may experience an overwhelming flood of maternal affection for your baby, wanting to cuddle and protect her, but don't be too surprised if all you feel like is a quick glance to make sure she's alright, then sit back exhausted wanting someone else to hold her and take care of her for you while you recover from the hard work of the past few hours. Also, you may feel a little overwhelmed at first by the responsibility of being a mother and you may be disappointed not to have felt the flood of maternal emotion that you may have expected.

A well-known children's doctor used to say there should be a sign in every delivery room saying "It won't necessarily be love at first sight. It may take time to fall in love with your baby". Try not to worry if you don't feel 'maternal' immediately – give it time, neither of you will benefit if you are feeling guilty or anxious about how you think you ought to be feeling.

Much has been written about the importance of bonding with your baby in the hours immediately following the birth. However, circumstances may arise that mean that you can't spend time with your baby immediately. She may need extra attention in the special care baby unit or you may have had a general anaesthetic. If she has a low APGAR score (this is a score given to babies at birth after observing their general condition, and gives an indication as to whether or not they will need any treatment) you may not be given her to hold straight away. This delay can be very disappointing and worrying after waiting so long.

Try not to worry too much – it doesn't mean that you will not be able to form a bond with your baby just because the opportunity to get to know her is delayed. When you finally hold your baby, you will have lots of time to get to know each other. You can spend time cuddling her, unwrapping her tightly curled arms and legs, looking at her and really believing she is here at last. She may clasp hold of your finger tightly and as you talk to her and gaze into each others eyes, you may wonder what to make of each other.

You may find that you are very emotional in the first few days. During pregnancy, your placenta produced large quantities of the hormone progesterone. Once the placenta has been delivered, the level of progesterone in your blood stream drops considerably and your highly emotional state may be partially due to this sudden fall in hormonal levels. It is also partly due to a reaction to the physical and emotional stresses of labour, as well as coming to terms with the dramatic physical changes in your body and the responsibility of becoming a mother. When you think about what you're having to cope with, it's no wonder your moods change erratically.

Because all your emotions seem very near the surface, it only takes something very minor to set you off. One minute you may be laughing hysterically with others over something you wouldn't normally find particularly funny and the next minute you may be moved to tears by something you have read or seen on television or something someone has said. You may find yourself over-reacting with feelings of anger or frustration or failure if someone appears to criticise your abilities as a mother, and if your partner is late at visiting time that can be the last straw.

For most women, this emotional see-saw, feeling up one minute and down the next, lasts only a few days and is often referred to as the baby blues.

Unfortunately, a very small percentage of women suffer from something more than the three day blues and need to be admitted to hospital for treatment of the severe form of postnatal illness called puerperal psychosis.

About one in ten women experience a less severe, but very real, depression which may last for months. In some cases, this depression does not begin until many weeks after the birth. It can be quite a shock to find yourself feeling constantly worn out and totally uninterested in everything around you, including your partner and your baby, just at a time in your life when you expected to feel happy and fulfilled. You may feel as if you are living in a shell, completely detached from those around you.

It is important to recognise this depression for what it is and take steps to deal with it rather than to just keep hoping that tomorrow you might snap out of it and feel better. Feelings of hopelessness and worthlessness, coupled with a complete lack of energy and enthusiasm for anything, which last for more than a few days can be significant signs of depression. These may be accomplished by overwhelming feelings of guilt, failure and loss of interest in sex, food and other people around you. You may also experience disturbed sleep patterns. Most people will be up and down from time to time in the early days. It's when the down lasts for days on end

> ❝I wish I'd known about the powerful hold on your emotions, even when I was trying to sleep.
>
> I decided not to have any extra help or visits for the first week at home. Just the four of us. It was a golden time and I would recommend that other relatives should be banned from visits for the first week.❞

that you and your partner should be aware of possible postnatal depression and seek help.

Do discuss honestly with your health visitor or GP how you are feeling, so that if you are suffering from postnatal depression you can be helped to recover from it as quickly as possible. One of the saddest facts about postnatal depression is that it is often not diagnosed until weeks after its onset. People often feel it is their fault and struggle on in the hope that they will get better.

Your doctor may prescribe a course of anti-depressant tablets which, unlike tranquillisers, are not addictive, although they do have side effects which are especially noticeable when you first start taking the tablets. Tell your doctor if you are breastfeeding so that he doesn't prescribe any drugs which might be harmful to your baby. Whatever you eat or drink comes through in minute quantities in your breast milk.

It is important to realise that there are also things you can do yourself to aid your recovery. Look at the suggestions on page 104 for dealing with stress. Many of them are just as successful for coping with depression. Talking to someone, trying to work out some very simple realistic goals for yourself and not taking on too much at any one time might help you. See if there is a self help group in your area, where mothers who have experienced postnatal depression get together to support each other (see addresses at the back of the book for more details).

Be realistic about how long it is likely to take to recover from postnatal depression and don't be too hard on yourself. Do the things that make you feel better and try to avoid the situations that make you feel worse. Take it in small manageable steps, one day at a time. Allow time for exercise and relaxation and enough time for your own meals so that you don't have to feel constantly rushed. Acknowledge that you are ill and need time to recover just as you would if you had flu or a broken leg. Recognising that you too have needs, allowing yourself to leave tasks that aren't essential and trying not to feel guilty about them are an important part of recovery.

THE FIRST FEW DAYS

If your baby was born at home, you may be feeling very happy and content, secure in familiar surroundings and able to make the decisions and choices about your baby's care which might be more difficult if you were in a hospital environment. On the other hand, if you had to campaign hard to get your wish to have your baby at home, you may find it difficult to admit to any negative feelings you might be experiencing about the birth or afterwards. Nothing is quite as we expect it to be, so try to be realistic – acknowledge and allow yourself those feelings, the negative as well as the positive.

It is very tempting, if you are feeling fit and well, to take up the reins of running the household again too soon. You will be surprised at how tired you can get looking after a young baby and if you try to do too much too soon, you will just get over-tired. You will never be able to recapture those first few days, so make the most of any offers of help that you have and allow yourself adequate time both to recover and to get to know your baby.

On the other hand, if your baby was born in hospital, you will probably find the first few days on a postnatal ward a strange mixture of experiences. There may be a great sense of

fun and sharing of new experiences with others in a similar situation where you are all learning together. You may be very reassured by the presence of experienced midwives who can offer support and advice on how to care for your new baby. Alternatively, you may be lonely and homesick, frustrated by the lack of privacy and the conflicting advice, and feel a failure as you struggle to learn how to cope with your baby surrounded by others who all seem far more knowing and confident than you. If you are very unhappy do speak to someone about it and if you feel that going home would be the solution for you, then you should go home. It does not matter if you are booked for a longer stay in the hospital, you can change your mind.

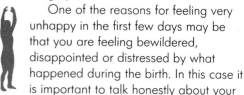

One of the reasons for feeling very unhappy in the first few days may be that you are feeling bewildered, disappointed or distressed by what happened during the birth. In this case it is important to talk honestly about your labour with someone who is a good listener. After any major life event, there is a need to talk through and re-live the experience over and over again. This seems to help get the many different aspects of any experience into perspective. Bottling up any negative feelings and pretending that everything is fine, will not be very helpful to you.

You may find that there are gaps where you can't quite remember what happened or why. Discussing the birth with someone who was with you, such as your partner or midwife, can be very helpful as they may be able to fill in the gaps for you. Everyone wants to share your excitement at the arrival of your new baby but it is especially important to be able to talk through the whole experience in a way that helps you to understand it. You may be able to talk to your antenatal teacher about your experience. She will probably have had a lot of experience of listening to women in these circumstances.

Many women who have had a difficult labour, or one in which they feel that they had no opportunity to make any decisions about their care, have a real need to talk through their experiences. If they don't have the opportunity to talk about it, or if they don't recognise the importance of being able to talk about it, they may expend a huge amount of emotional energy in the early months, reliving the experience in their own minds or just trying to forget about it. Over the years, I have come across a number of such women who, years later, are still trying to come to terms with what happened during the birth of their first baby and may find that it is still affecting them, especially when they become pregnant again.

Your partner will also benefit from being able to share his feelings about the whole experience. You may find that writing it all down is a useful way of getting things into perspective and perhaps recognising that there were positive as well as negative aspects to it. If you feel the need for more explanation about anything that occurred during the birth, write to the general manager at the hospital in which you had your baby, or ask to see the director of midwifery services or your consultant. Your local Community Health Council should be able to help you if you wish to make a complaint. It may be very important to you in any future pregnancy to understand what happened and why during this labour. Do write too, if you felt that your experience and the care you received was very good. It is so important for midwives to get feedback on what women find helpful in making labour a positive experience for them.

The ability to communicate how you are feeling, whether positive or negative, is an important part of dealing with the stresses in everyday life, and will stand you in good stead during your years as a parent.

• • • • • •

THE NEW FAMILY

The arrival of a new baby is an exciting time for any couple. They can learn together how to care for their new baby and share the joys and pleasures, but it may seem quite a daunting responsibility at first. Being at home with your baby you will be able to respond much more spontaneously and individually to your baby's needs than you could possibly do in hospital, but there are bound to be moments of anxiety once you are on your own. There will be times when you don't know why your baby is crying and that can be very frustrating and scary. However, you will soon get to know your baby, and what she needs, if you allow yourself to relax and believe that your instincts can be relied upon.

One of the things that most new mothers find difficult to cope with is the conflicting advice that they receive from well meaning people all around them. People always tend to give advice as if their way is the only and 'right' way to do something. Of course this isn't the case. We are all individuals and so are our babies and what will be right for one family simply will not suit another. Listen to what people have to say, because there may be something useful you can learn from their experience, choose whatever aspects of their advice seems to be right for you and your family and politely discard anything you feel instinctively won't be right for you.

Some of the difficulties of adjusting to life at home as a new mother result from the way in which your new role is seen by you and by other people.

Ann Oakley in her book *The Sociology of Housework* talks about the way in which housework is regarded as a natural part of being a woman but is not regarded as 'real work' because it is unpaid and done in the privacy of the home. It seems strange that the same jobs, done for someone else would be regarded as worthwhile paid employment.

There is a perception in society that a woman at home has a great deal of freedom and choice. It seems as if she is not bound by the time restraints and supervision of an employer and therefore must have endless opportunity for indulging in anything that interests her. In reality, a mother at home may not see herself as having any choice about what she does. She feels she ought to be doing all sorts of things for her family which leave her with very little time for herself.

There is often a sense at the end of the day of being exhausted yet feeling that you have achieved very little and what you have achieved will all need to be done again tomorrow. The boredom and monotony of many household chores, which are repeated daily without a break from them even at weekends, can be very stressful.

It is often assumed that motherhood is a natural role which a woman is instinctively good at and it can be quite demoralising to find yourself failing to live up to the image of the mother you thought you could be. If only it were recognised that it is a role which needs skills like any other job, skills which need to be learnt and developed through experience and making mistakes. Feelings of self-worth and self-esteem are normally closely tied up with our work and the value society places upon it.

Many people underestimate the variety of skills needed to be a mother and run a home successfully, so it is all too easy to feel undervalued and overworked, which in turn leads to low self-esteem and lack of confidence.

In many families today, the father plays a

> **❝I do occasionally get fed up with the increased volume of chores that I find myself doing. There has definitely been a shift in balance of chore-doing between my husband and myself which goes beyond the fact that I am at home all day making more mess.❞**

much bigger role in caring for the baby and older children, and doing his share of the housework, than in previous generations, though these situations are not very common. However, even when a mother is also in paid employment, it is still she who does the major share of all the childcare and household chores even though she is in full-time paid employment. In one recent survey called 'Inside the Family: Changing roles of men and women', it was found that, on average, the tasks involved in looking after a child (especially under the age of two) took just over seven hours a day. By far the greatest part of the childcare tasks were performed by the mother. It was interesting to note that the father's involvement tended to be concentrated on the more enjoyable and less demanding aspects of child care, such as outings and playtime. In other words, the fathers took little routine responsibility for their children but were seen to be very involved because they took the children out and spent time playing with them.

This may lead to feelings of resentment between the two partners. She resents the fact that her partner can escape from the pressures of the home and have the stimulating company of other adults and it seems that his life has hardly changed at all. On the other hand, he may feel resentful of the fact that he is now the sole breadwinner having to hold down a demanding job when he may be feeling very tired after sleepless nights. He may also feel jealous of the close relationship his partner has with the baby and the time she can spend with her. He may feel that she has the easier option with time to herself at home and the time to spend with their baby, unaware of the true nature of the demands placed upon her by being at home with a small baby all day.

In some families the mother and father have switched the traditional roles and he stays at home to look after the baby while she goes out to work.

In reality, it is very difficult to make time for yourself when coping with the numerous complicated and exhausting tasks of being a mum and running a home. It is important that you and your partner are able to share these feelings with each other before they get out of proportion. If left, it becomes harder to discuss them for fear of hurting each other's feelings. This may be the time when you both need extra love and caring, but because of tiredness and trying to meet the needs of your new baby, you may both find providing that extra caring extremely difficult.

DEVELOPING YOUR RELATIONSHIP WITH YOUR PARTNER

It is well worth making the effort to spend time alone together – arrange for someone to babysit, even if just for an hour or so, when the baby is quite young. Arrange with another mother if you have no family nearby, that you look after her baby for her while she and her partner go out and vice versa. You will probably find it surprisingly hard to leave your baby the first time but it is important to recognise that you and your partner still have a life together, quite independent of your other role as parents.

You will need to work out a balance which is right for you between caring for your baby and any other children you have and continuing to develop your relationship with your partner.

For many couples the first few months as parents can be extremely tiring, frustrating and demanding and for many it can be a time of arguments and rows, as each tries to get what he or she needs from the other at a time when both have least to give. Recognising that it is going to be hard and will take time to adjust to, may be the first step to solving many of the problems. Being honest about how you are each feeling and trying to work out solutions together is much healthier than pretending everything is fine when deep down you are boiling with resentment. Many couples find that pregnancy and parenthood provide a real opportunity to strengthen and deepen their relationship. Becoming a parent often brings out a tenderness and an awareness of themselves and others which they hadn't recognised before and often brings them closer together as a couple.

Lack of sleep can make even the smallest of problems seem insurmountable and this tiredness often leads to feelings of resentment and lack of communication between couples. This, in turn can lead to problems with your sex life. The spontaneity you used to enjoy may be temporarily altered if the baby cries at the wrong moment, or if one of you feels too tired just when the other is aroused and wanting to make love.

If you don't always feel like intercourse, there are other ways of communicating and demonstrating your love for each other, rather than letting it become a major problem between the two of you. During the months of pregnancy you have not had to worry about contraception. You will now need to use some form of contraception if you don't want to become pregnant again. It is possible to become pregnant within a month or two of the birth of your baby and although breastfeeding on an unrestricted basis does reduce the chances of becoming pregnant, it is not a foolproof method of contraception.

You can resume intercourse as soon after your baby's birth as you feel you want to. You may then suddenly be aware that you have not thought about what contraceptive methods you are going to use. Ideally it is worth discussing this before the birth as once the baby arrives you have such a lot to think about. You may need to change the type of contraceptive you used before the birth. The NCT has a leaflet on *Sex in Pregnancy and After Birth* which is available from NCT Maternity Sales.

YOUR OLDER CHILD

A new baby in the family is a very exciting time for older brothers and sisters. Children are usually fascinated by babies. As the baby grows and begins to recognise and respond to those around her, it is lovely to see the gurgles of delight from the baby when she sees her older brother or sister and the pleasure that the older child gets. He may keep the baby happily occupied for ages while she sits and watches him playing, although he may get a little frustrated when she is not able to join in with his games. It is quite hard, when you are very young, to understand that babies coo and gurgle and don't seem to be able to make fire engine or bear noises like you can.

As a mother with a new baby and an older child or children, you may feel constantly torn between the demands of the baby and your other child or children.

Most children will take a little while to adjust to the new member of the family. Some will seem to cope very happily with no real problems, but others may find it hard to adjust to a new baby. Be on the look out for a change in their eating, sleeping patterns or their general behaviour, which may indicate that they are finding it hard to adjust. Older children are less dependent on you than a very young child and they are able to talk about how they are feeling if you encourage them to, so any problems that do arise may be easier to handle than when the other child is very

young. In the majority of families the older child is likely to be under the age of five when the new baby arrives.

For a toddler the adjustment may be more difficult. He may suddenly become very clingy and more dependent. This sort of behaviour is quite usual. The arrival of a new baby means he is having to cope with some major changes in his life which up to now has probably been very safe and settled in a comfortable, familiar routine. If your baby was born in hospital, your child has also had to cope with being separated from you for a few days.

During the pregnancy, he was probably aware that you were somehow different, growing larger and getting more tired and perhaps unable to run and kick a ball or get down on the floor to play with him as you used to. Once the baby is born it will be hard to find the time to play with him as the baby takes up so much of your time.

However much you tried to prepare him for the arrival of a new baby, it is bound to be strange at first and he will take some time to make the necessary adjustments. There are many different ways in which his feelings may become apparent.

You may find that he regresses to waking at night, or wanting to go back into nappies just like the baby; he may be very aggressive towards you or the baby; he might be more tearful than usual or suddenly become quite naughty, deliberately doing things you ask him not to do, or become very possessive with his toys which can lead to tantrums at playschool or when playing with friends. It is hard to be patient if you are feeling tired and irritable from lack of sleep, and your toddler is trying to get your attention by doing awful things which he never did before, like drawing on the walls. He may feel that any attention from you, even if you are cross with him, is better than when you don't seem to notice him at all because you are too preoccupied with the baby or too tired.

It can be very difficult to keep calm in the middle of the night when you have just managed to get back to sleep after feeding the baby and your toddler wakes with a wet bed. Don't be too hard on him. It is not uncommon for small children to go back to wetting the bed or waking at night after the arrival of a sister or brother.

Try to understand that this behaviour is all part of his feelings of confusion and insecurity. He is trying to get used to not being the centre of attention any more and learning how to share you with someone else. Someone once said, "Try and think how you would react if your partner came home one evening with another woman and said 'I still love you just as much as ever darling but I'd like to introduce you to someone else I love who is coming to live with us.'" Most of us would find that situation difficult to adjust to.

No matter how rarely you seem to find the opportunity, when you are able to devote some time to your toddler listen to him and take a real interest in what he is doing. For example, if he shows you a drawing or a painting that he has done, comment in detail on the colours and shapes and discuss it with him rather than just saying 'what a nice painting'. If he is describing something to you, let him take his time and get down to his level and listen and watch carefully. If you can give him warning some time before you are going to have to stop playing with him or when it is lunchtime, there will be less tendency for him to feel cheated at having his game stopped just when it was getting interesting.

❝He's taken to waking up at night since the twins arrived and coming into our bed. Some nights we end up with all of them in the bed together. I have come home from night duty to find all of them in the bed, mum, the twins and the two boys so I have to go and sleep in one of the boy's bunk beds.❞

Encouraging his co-operation without a constant battle of wills and tears of frustration on his part and angry words on yours, takes a good deal of patience and ingenuity, especially if he is behaving in an aggressive way. At the end of a long and tiring day it can be quite hard to think creatively about how to avoid tantrums, but with practice it gets easier.

Try making a game out of things that need to be done, like tidying up. 'Shall we see if you can collect more toys than me to put in your toy box before we go and have your bath' or give him a choice between two options, both of which will achieve what you want him to do. This may encourage his co-operation and be enjoyable for you both. For example, try saying 'It's bathtime. Do you want to chase me up to the bathroom or shall I chase you tonight.' This probably means you end up with him in the bath as you wanted and both of you with a fit of the giggles.

Before you sit down to feed the baby, get everything your child might need, like a drink, potty, books or games by your side, then you won't find yourself leaping up and down all the time. Choose somewhere with enough space for all three of you to sit comfortably, then you can physically relax and put your feet up. Feedtimes for the baby can become a special time for your toddler when you read to him, do puzzles or tell him stories. The baby is unlikely to notice that she doesn't have your full attention providing she is getting the milk she needs. Your toddler may feel less resentful towards the baby if he sees her feedtimes as a special time to be with you. There are bound to be times when you can feed the baby alone and enjoy getting to know her, away from the demands of your toddler.

If you can keep the pattern of his life as familiar as possible, the changes he has to face will be minimised. Provided this in itself does not become too stressful for you, it may make life easier all round. For example, most babies will cope quite happily with having a short feed before dashing off to playgroup and then returning home to finish off that feed half an hour later.

You could try bathing them both together. Get everything you need ready before you start and just give the baby a quick dip in the toddler's bath water, then you can dress and feed her in the bathroom while keeping an eye on your toddler as he plays in the bath. She will then probably sleep or sit and watch you while you wash, dry and dress him. It might help if your partner could hold the baby while you spend time reading to your toddler and giving him some time which is his own.

Time is something mothers always seem to be short of. It is all too easy to fall into the 'Yes in a minute darling' syndrome while we dash about trying to fit in all the household chores that always seem to need doing. Children grow up very quickly and before you know what has happened they are off to school while the housework will still be there.

It is impossible to do everything around the house yourself and have plenty of time for the children. Don't try to be a superwoman. Look after the people first and the things second. Don't forget yourself and remember – children are very resilient.

Decide on your priorities and work out a pattern that suits you and your family situation.

James age 2 years, brother of Emily aged 4 months.

❝Mummy, mummy, I just had a double decker bath. Daddy put Emily in the big bath with me!!!❞

If having a tidy, clean house is very important to you, perhaps you can afford to get someone in to help you occasionally. If not, you will need to negotiate with your partner and get him to agree to do some of the routine chores, allowing you time for play, or outings with your toddler, or time for yourself. If may help to work out between you a way of dividing up the jobs that you both consider essential rather than trying to fit it all in to your busy day and feeling guilty and exhausted by the evening, or just ending up with a situation where you are doing all the mundane household chores while your partner takes on the pleasurable childcare tasks.

Make a list of all the things that need to be done, including the childcare tasks like feeding, bathing and changing nappies, the household chores, as well as things like time for each other, hobbies, time with the older child etc. Sit down with your partner and decide who shall do what and when. Discuss whether or not you take it for granted that certain tasks are the sole responsibility of one or other partner. Discussing together what being a mum or a dad means to each of you can be a very enlightening exercise.

Do accept help from friends who offer to take your baby or toddler out so that you can rest. It is also nice to be able to go out alone with your older child while someone else looks after the baby. This may be a time when he can have a few new privileges and try out some new activities if it seems to be of benefit to him. If he seems very unhappy with a new situation, like playschool for example, you may need to decide whether it might be better to stop going and try again when he is more settled.

Finding time to enjoy the positive side of motherhood, the fun and the laughter, amidst the hundred and one things that always seem to need doing, is not easy, especially when you feel constantly tired but the benefits to you and your children will far outweigh the disadvantages of not always having all the jobs done on time.

> I hope my children
> Look back on today
> And see a mother
> Who had time to play
> There will be years
> For cleaning and cooking
> Children grow up
> When you're not looking
> So quiet down cobwebs
> Dust go to sleep
> I'm rocking my baby
> And babies don't keep

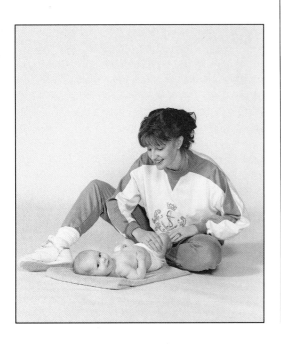

COPING WITH THE DEMANDS OF BEING A MOTHER

For most mothers, motherhood is very rewarding – seeing their baby thrive and develop gives them their greatest satisfaction in life, but the demands can be very stressful.

Stress occurs when you feel that the demands made upon you exceed your ability to manage them. Many different factors influence your ability to cope with any given situation – personality, past experience and upbringing all affect the way you respond to a situation. Others may respond very differently in a similar situation. Deadlines bring out the best in some people, challenging them and stimulating them while they cause sheer panic in others.

Stress can affect the body, mind and the emotions. It's symptoms include:

- Feeling helpless
- Feeling panicky
- Feeling insecure and unable to cope
- Feeling angry and frustrated
- Feeling anxious and keyed-up
- Feeling fearful and worried
- Feeling bored and apathetic
- Lack of concentration
- Loss of a sense of proportion
- Forgetfulness
- Short-tempered
- Can't think straight
- More minor accidents and mistakes
- Sweaty palms
- Dry mouth
- Slight feeling of breathlessness
- Muscle tension and headaches
- Heart pounding
- Butterflies in the stomach
- Altered sleeping patterns
- Cold hands and feet
- Can't sit still
- Clenched jaw

Research shows that the dominant characteristics of people who seem able to withstand stress are that they regard change as a challenge and not as a threat and they believe that they are able to exercise some control over a situation. They are realistic about a situation, seeing it as it is, not as they would like it to be, and they tend to take a positive approach and try not to imagine the worst. They take responsibility for themselves and are able to cope with disappointment if it occurs.

> 66 Be prepared to ask for what you need rather than struggling on getting horribly frustrated. I suppose it depends on your personality whether or not you can easily ask for help. 99

Other factors also influence how you cope with a situation. Having adequate information about a situation will help you to realise what may be required in terms of time, energy or skills to deal with it and it certainly helps decision making if you have all the facts available. In a new or worrying situation good information is particularly important.

The number of existing demands already being made on your time will also affect the way you respond to any new demand – you can only handle so much at any one time. This may mean that you sometimes have to say no to someone. Learning to do so without feeling guilty is very important. Being able to admit that you can't take on something is not a sign of weakness or failure but a sign of honest and realistic acceptance of your abilities and limitations. Asking for help shows that you value support and may in turn enable someone else to recognise that it is okay to ask for help. Many people cause their own stress by having very high expectations of themselves and setting unrealistic personal goals for themselves.

Your mental and physical health is also significant. When you are not 100% fit, you need to slow down so that you have the extra energy available to get well again. Struggling on, gallantly trying to cope with physical and mental fatigue, or illness, as well as all the other demands can lead to chronic fatigue, mood swings and misery for everyone.

Some factors may be completely outside your control. It is important to recognise and accept those that are, and concentrate instead on any others which you may be able to alter. There is an old prayer that may be helpful in this context, which says:

> 'God grant me the strength to change the things I can change, the courage to accept the things that I cannot change and the wisdom to know the difference.'

THE A B C OF MANAGING STRESS

You may think it is impossible to change the way you are but, by following this A B C of managing stress, you can change the way you respond to demands made upon you.

A is for Awareness. This means being able to recognise the specific causes of your stress (sometimes called stressors), knowing how you react to the demands and recognising the symptoms when you begin to feel overloaded with demands.

B is for Balance. Too little stimulus or challenge can be as stressful as too much. You need just enough to motivate and stimulate you, without putting you under too much pressure. If you can become aware of the causes of stress and achieve the right balance of stimulus you can control the stress.

C is the Control. Recognise what causes you stress. Choosing when and how many demands you will accept, as well as the way you respond to those different demands, will enable you to take control.

Awareness: The first step to dealing with stress is identifying the cause. Try to be very specific. Instead of saying 'It's this house that is causing my stress', try to identify what it is about the house that is making you feel stressed. Is it that you feel that you haven't got enough room now you have a baby? Are you worried about the mortgage repayments? Is there damp in the baby's bedroom that makes you concerned about his health?

Once you have identified exactly what it is, you can begin to look at it and discuss with your partner ways of tackling the problem. It may be that what you regard as a major source of worry, your partner does not see as such. It is important that you both acknowledge that what seems to be a worry to one of you is very real and needs dealing with, not dismissing as trivial. More information or help about the subject from outside sources may help you to deal with a situation more effectively, or, alternatively, it may help you to put it in perspective and realise that it isn't as much of a problem as you thought it was.

When the body perceives a threat or danger, many physiological changes occur which prepare the body for action. This is known as 'the fight or flight response' and it is a very important factor in ensuring survival in a real danger situation. The body produces hormones which cause the heart rate and breathing to increase to get more oxygen to the muscles quickly. Sweating increases to cool the body down, blood is diverted to the muscles ready for quick action in fighting or fleeing from the danger and the liver releases sugar, cholesterol and fatty acids into the blood stream so that they can supply a ready source of energy to the muscles.

In a situation where we are required to physically fight or flee, the body uses up all this ready energy and is quickly restored to normal. For most of us, usually, any threat or danger is likely to be imagined and not real. Constant worry and anxiety about something will produce a similar stress response to that which occurs with 'the fight or flight response'. The problem is that it is likely to be a longer-term situation and the body has no means of discharging the extra energy and tension and so has difficulty getting back to normal. Living life on a day-to-day basis in this highly charged, ready-to-explode state is neither helpful nor healthy. It is important to be able to recognise when we are getting into that state and to know how to relax and unwind and get back to normal.

Balance: Discovering your optimum stress level means looking at what you do and whether or not there is a balance in your life between the tasks that are essential, even though they may be boring, and activities you enjoy. By making time for enjoyable activities, you will gain renewed energy to help you cope with the less rewarding tasks that need to be done every day.

An extremely useful exercise is to write out a list of all the different tasks you do in a 24 hour period, breaking the day into 30 minute intervals. For example:

5.00am . . . Fed baby
5.30am . . . Back to sleep
6.00am . . . .
6.30am . . . Toddler woke up
7.00am . . . Breakfast for toddler, put washing in machine
7.30am . . . Washed up dishes, fed baby
8.00am . . . .
8.30am . . . .
9.00am . . . .

When you have completed the list go through it and underline all the things you did that you really enjoyed and circle the ones you find boring, repetitive and monotonous. Look at your list and see if there is any balance between the two types of activities. Was there anywhere in the day when you had some time entirely to yourself and did something which didn't require you to be giving of your time and energy to other people.

By identifying some of the stressors in your life, you can see where you could make changes in order to allow some space for yourself and it may be a useful basis for discussion and negotiation with your partner. It will be very hard for him to underestimate all that you do each day when it is clearly set down in black and white in front of you both.

He could fill in a similar chart for his day and then you could discuss how you share out the tasks that need to be done. It might be helpful to decide which ones are essential, which are important, and which ones you could leave for another time or perhaps ask someone else to do for you.

Control: It may be that you need to take control of a stressful situation by avoiding it or changing it if possible. However, it is more likely that the way to exercise some sort of control is to take responsibility for getting what you need and asking clearly for it.

Make sure that you allow time for exercise and relaxation in your life and try to develop some positive actions and attitudes with which to tackle stressful situations, such as the examples given below.

• **Talk things through.** It can be a great relief to share a problem with someone you trust or in a group such as at an NCT postnatal exercise class. Simply talking about the situation often puts it in perspective.

• **Write it down.** This helps you to see the problem more clearly.

• **Sort it out.** Make a list of some practical options and then choose the alternative that

seems the most appropriate one for your particular situation.

• **Work it off.** Do something physical, like going for a bike ride, a swim or a walk, to take your mind off the problem.

• **Delay it.** Set aside a specific time later in the day or week for thinking things through without other distractions.

• **Breathe it away.** Take a deep breath and as you sigh out, try to relax as many muscles as you possibly can.

• **Distance it.** Imagine yourself in a few weeks or years time – how important will this problem seem then.

• **Exaggerate it.** Think about the worst that could possibly happen in this particular situation. Is it very likely?

• **Balance it.** Think about any positive aspects to the situation and be glad of those, rather than just thinking about the negative side of the problem.

• **Laugh it off.** Smile and try to see the funny side of the situation.

REST

As a mother with a small baby and perhaps a toddler as well, the one thing you will be short of is sleep. Small babies need frequent feeds so you should anticipate being woken up a number of times a night in the early weeks. There is no magic age when your baby will sleep through the night, it will happen when she is ready to, so you need to make sure that you cope with this period of her life with the minimum stress to you and your partner. If you were working at a job which required you to work at night, you would think nothing of sleeping for a part of the day to make up for the lack of sleep.

It is amazing how many mothers spend many hours of the night awake, dealing with a baby or small child and then expect to carry on as normal during the day.

You might have six or seven hours of sleep but if it has been interrupted every hour or so, you will probably feel as if you have had hardly any sleep at all. Do try to make time to rest during the day while your baby is still feeding at night. If you have a toddler, you could coincide your rest with his sleep or his favourite TV or radio programme or story tape.

Fatigue is a major contributing factor in postnatal depression and is something to be avoided. Don't fall into the trap of dashing about, fitting in odd chores every time the baby is asleep. If you can rest in the middle of the day, you are less likely to feel hassled and tearful over the evening meal. You could try going to bed very early some evenings and your partner could change the baby and bring her to you in bed for a late feed and then settle her down again. You can go straight back to sleep for a few hours before the next feed in the early hours of the morning.

> **❝One of the most helpful things when I had postnatal depression was being able to talk to some close friends who understood.❞**

RELAXATION

Relaxation is a very useful skill to acquire and one that has very positive and measurable effects in tackling the symptoms of stress. When someone is very relaxed their brain waves, heart rate and breathing slow down and all the effects of the stress response are reversed. It takes practice to be able to relax effectively, but it is a skill anyone can master. It isn't just something you do when lying down in a dark and quiet room – once you have learnt how to relax you should be able to use it in any situation to minimise the tension in your muscles.

Initially when learning how to relax, set aside time when you are not likely to be interrupted or distracted. Wear comfortable clothing and make sure you are warm enough. Sit well back in a chair with your back supported and your feet resting on the floor. If your feet do not reach the floor put them on a telephone directory, or something similar, so that your thigh muscles are relaxed. Let your legs roll outwards from your hips and wriggle your toes to release tension. Rest your hands on your lap with your elbows comfortably by your side and your fingers slightly separated and gently curved.

If your head is not supported by the back of the chair, make sure it is well-balanced on your shoulders, not tilted too far back or with your chin poking too far forward. Let your eyelids droop and close if that feels comfortable for you. Become aware of the places where your body is touching and receiving support from the chair and the floor. Sigh out and let yourself sink down into that support.

Without trying to alter it in any way, become aware of your breathing. The slow gentle rise of the abdomen and chest as you breathe in and the fall of the chest and abdomen as you breathe out. Be aware that it is the out breath which is the relaxation phase of breathing. Focus on the breath out and use this to help you get rid of any unnecessary tension that still remains. Each time you sigh out, think of letting go a little more and sinking down into the support.

As you breathe out you will become aware of a slight pause before the next in breath. Allow the pause and then let the breath in take care of itself.

Check through the body again – think about easing the shoulders down away from your ears and making your neck a little longer, check that your legs are rolled outwards from the hips, allow your abdomen to go soft and just sit quietly and enjoy the feeling of peace and calm spreading through your body. If any part of your body is not comfortable, move it slightly and sigh out and ease away the tension from that part, sinking down into the support of the chair. After a short while, wriggle your toes and fingers, stretch or yawn if you need to and then when you are ready, open your eyes. Don't try to relax for too long at first, especially if you get fidgety after a short time. As you get better at it, you will be able to relax more quickly and for longer periods.

There are many different methods of relaxation and it is important to find a method that works for you. If you find it hard to get the feel of relaxing and easing away of tension from the muscles as described above, you can try the more specific technique described below.

Registering the Feeling of Tension

Tighten any group of muscles in the body as hard as you possibly can and register that feeling of MAXIMUM tension, then release the tension and recognise the difference. Then try tensing the muscles a moderate amount and register MODERATE tension, then release. Lastly, try tensing the muscles with the barest MINIMUM of tension, recognise what that feels like and then release. Learning how to recognise different levels of tension will help you to learn how to let go.

Tension Releasing Exercises

Work through the different large muscle groups of the body as follows. With each group you will need to tense the muscles three times – first using MAXIMUM (MAX), then MODERATE (MOD) and then MINIMUM (MIN) tension, releasing them fully in between and thinking carefully about how it feels each time. Make sure that you fully release all

tension from the muscles after the last tensing.

Most of the following exercises can be done sitting up or lying down. If lying down causes a strain, try placing either a cushion or a rolled towel under your thighs so that your knees are just slightly bent.

Face Muscles

Purse your lips together as if you were trying to make the sound 'O'. Feel the tension around the mouth, then release. (MAX, MOD and MIN tension.)

Screw up your eyes as if squinting in bright sunlight. Register the feeling of tension around your eyes, then release. (MAX, MOD and MIN tension.)

Clench your teeth together and register the feeling of tension around the temples and the jaw, then release. (MAX, MOD and MIN tension.)

Shoulder and Chest Muscles

Press your elbows against the side of your body and register the tension across the chest and shoulders, then release. (MAX, MOD and MIN tension.)

Shrug both your shoulders up towards your ears and register the feeling of tension in your muscles on the top of the shoulders and also up the sides of your neck, then release. (MAX, MOD and MIN tension.)

Back of Upper Arm Muscles

Press the back of your wrist against the top of your thigh or against the floor or chair. Register the feeling of tension in the back of the upper arms, then release. (MAX, MOD and MIN tension.)

Front of the Upper Arm Muscles

Place your hand underneath your thigh and try to lift your hand against the resistance of your body. Register the tension in the front of the upper arms, then release. (MAX MOD and MIN tension.)

Back of Forearm Muscles

Keeping the wrist in contact with your thighs or the arm of the chair, raise your hand off the surface and feel the tension in the back of the hand and forearm, then release. (MAX, MOD and MIN tension.)

Front of Forearm Muscles

Press your fingertips firmly down onto your thigh or the arm of the chair, making your hand into the shape of a spider. Feel the tension in your forearm, then release. (MAX, MOD and MIN tension.)

Neck Muscles

Press the back of your head firmly into the floor, being careful to keep your chin tucked in. Feel the tension in the back of the neck, then release. (MAX, MOD and MIN tension.)

If you prefer, it is also possible to press the head back without it being in contact with any surface and get the feeling of tension and release when you are sitting with your head unsupported.

Back Muscles

Arch the small of your back away from the floor or chair, increasing the distance between your waistband and the floor or chair until you feel the tension, then release. (MAX, MOD and MIN tension.)

Abdominal Muscles

Pull in your abdominal muscles as if you are trying to do up a belt that is too small for you. Feel the tension, then release. (MAX, MOD and MIN tension.)

. . . . . .

Thigh Muscles

Press the backs of your knees firmly down against the floor. Feel the tension in the front of your thighs, then release. (MAX, MOD and MIN tension.) If you are sitting, you will need to press your feet into the ground and try to slide your legs straight out in front of you to feel the tension.

Squeeze your thighs together and feel the tension in the inner thigh muscles, then release and let the legs roll apart. (MAX, MOD and MIN tension.)

Lower Leg Muscles

Point your toes, extending the ankle joints at the same time. Feel the tension in your calf muscles (be careful not to point too hard or you may give yourself cramp). Release the tension. (MAX, MOD and MIN tension.)

Pull your toes up towards you and flex the ankle joints. Feel the tension up the front of the lower legs, then release. (MAX, MOD and MIN tension.)

After the exercises

Once you have worked your way through the different muscle groups, check that your breathing is calm and rhythmical and that your whole body feels relaxed and comfortable as you sigh out and release any hidden tension. Sit or lie still for a few minutes, enjoying the feeling you have created within your body before wriggling and stretching. If you have been lying down to relax, make sure you get up very carefully. Turn onto your side, then slowly push yourself up into a sitting position and then into an all-fours kneeling position. Place one foot in front of you on the ground in a half-kneeling position with your hands resting on the bent thigh. Push yourself up into a standing position.

VISUALISATION

This is a technique to aid relaxation. There is nothing mystical or magical about visualisation – it is part of the thinking process. We all make images or pictures when we think. Many people find that they are able to relax their bodies, but then find that their mind is working overtime and so they are not fully able to relax and unwind. Being able to calm your mind is very useful. One useful practical tip is to have a notepad and pen available when you settle down to relax, so that any thoughts that pop into your mind can be jotted down. Once you know that you don't have to keep trying to remember something, you can usually stop worrying about it.

Once you have worked through whatever kind of relaxation you have chosen to remove tension from your body, try the following technique to still the mind. The muscles which move the eyes are involved in the visualisation aspect of thinking, so being able to recognise tension in those little eye muscles and then learning to release that tension will enable you to quieten an active mind. If you wear contact lenses, you may find it more comfortable to remove them before starting this exercise.

Have your eyes open and keep your head still so that you only move your eyes. Look towards your right ear, hold for a second and recognise the tension in the eye muscles, then feel the eye muscles relax as you let your eyes return to look straight ahead. Repeat, this time looking to the left side.

Look up towards your eyebrows, feel the tension, then release. Look down towards your chin and feel the tension, then release.

Move your eyes quickly to the right, left, up and down, noticing the slight tension.

Focus on a spot a few feet away directly in front of you, just below eye level, and recognise that that is a relaxed position for the eye muscles. Check that your breathing is calm and rhythmical and if your eyelids feel heavy let them close, but still try to visualise the spot in front of you. Your eye muscles should be relaxed and it should be difficult to visualise anything else.

Some people like to visualise in great detail a place where they like being, such as a garden or the beach. They find that imagining the sights and sounds of that place allows them to fully relax and keeps their mind from racing and worrying. Others find that music helps them to relax. Use whatever particular visualisation method works best for you.

ECONOMY OF EFFORT

Relaxation is not just something you might be able to squeeze in for 5 minutes a day if you are lucky. Once you have learned the basic skill of relaxation and tension awareness, it is important that you try to use it whatever you are doing. If you are bending over changing the baby, sitting and feeding her, cooking the supper or watching television, get into the habit of checking your posture and looking for any signs of unnecessary tension. It is not essential to have your shoulders up under your ears and your hands gripping the steering wheel tightly when driving just because you are late. That unnecessary tension is very tiring and the more you can become aware of it and get rid of it the better you will feel.

TIME FOR YOURSELF

There are only so many hours in a day and trying to find the time to fit in all that needs to be done is a constant battle. Many a mother feels that time to herself, even to get a haircut or put on any make-up, is a luxury she cannot afford with all the demands her family make on her time. It's as if her own identity has been completely submerged beneath the new role of mothering and she feels that she is expected to work tirelessly and selflessly for years for her children. This can lead to feelings of frustration, resentment and guilt, and for some women undermines their confidence in their abilities to do anything other than mothering and housework. It is much healthier all round to recognise from the start that you have needs as well as your children and your partner and that it is not selfish to want some time to yourself.

FEELING COMFORTABLE

It is important to wear clothes that are easy to care for, comfortable, with easy access for breastfeeding, and washable as young babies and children have a habit of being sick or placing sticky marks on your clothes at frequent intervals. You may still be a little overweight following the pregnancy so it is important to choose clothes that don't exaggerate that fact.

Set aside some time, perhaps with a friend, to go through your wardrobe and find all the clothes that you can fit into and that you feel good in. Remember it is likely to be some months before you are completely back to your pre-pregnant size and shape. You may feel it is worth buying some new clothes that you can fit into now, rather than squeezing yourself into

TEN POINT PLAN FOR SUCCESSFULLY MANAGING STRESS

1 Identify the sources. Be specific about what is causing the stress, whether it be relationships, change, environment, finance etc.

2 Know yourself. How you respond to stress; acknowledge your true feelings.

3 Be prepared to change. It involves risk, but not being prepared to attempt change signals acceptance of the situation as it is.

4 Be assertive. Assertiveness means a) acknowledging your rights as well as the rights of the others, b) recognising your own needs as a woman, irrespective of your role as wife, mother, lover, daughter, c) allowing yourself the right to make mistakes and to enjoy your successes, d) asking clearly for what you want rather than hoping someone will notice, e) making clear your feelings.

5 Develop a positive approach. Don't expect the worst, imagine yourself winning through.

6 Make time for yourself. 'If I had more time to myself I would . . .' Write this out and fill in what you would do. Then look at your time sheet and see where you could find the time.

7 Learn to relax. Allow yourself time to practise so that you get better and better. Recognise tension in everyday activities and try to minimise it.

8 Take regular exercise. You will sleep better and feel better able to tackle the demands of the day.

9 Eat regular sensible meals. Don't consume high fat and sugary snacks while on the run.

10 Work out priorities. Set yourself realistic, achievable goals.

jeans that are tight and will hamper your circulation, make you feel uncomfortable and probably make you look larger than you actually are.

Skirts and trousers with tops and jumpers are usually easier than dresses while you are breastfeeding. Shortage of money for yourself now that you are no longer working is something you need to sort out with your partner. You may be able to treat yourself to something new and not too expensive, like some brightly coloured tops to team with and jazz up your existing wardrobe.

LOOKING GOOD

If wearing make-up makes you feel good and is important to you, then try to keep it simple so that you are able to find time to put on your make-up in the morning with a quick touch-up before you go out anywhere. If on the other hand, it is just one more chore that you haven't got time for then don't bother.

Cleansing and moisturising are an important part of good looking skin, so try to make sure that you don't flop into bed in exhaustion every night without paying some attention to your face. Eating sensibly and having enough sleep or relaxation are also important factors in looking good. Paying attention to those aspects of your life will inevitably have an effect on the way you look.

If you feel that a new, more easily manageable hair style is needed now that you have less time, discuss with your hairdresser the best style to suit you. Massaging your scalp is a wonderful way of releasing tension and should help to improve the circulation and condition of your hair. Use little circular movements with the fingertips, like kneading dough.

One of the most positive ways of looking good is to feel relaxed and happy, not stressed, anxious and guilt ridden. Making time for yourself and doing something you enjoy will put back lost energy and enable you to cope with this demanding new role.

Once you know your new baby and her patterns of feeding and sleeping, you may feel able to leave her in a creche or with a trusted friend or family member while you develop some new hobby or interest or study some new subject at evening classes. Rather than being bad for your baby or toddler, it is all part of the important lesson of learning to gradually become independent of you. It will be far less traumatic when she has to go to playgroup or start school if she has already got used to the idea that you aren't always by her side. Having a break from the constant demands of childcare can make a very positive contribution to the mother's emotional and mental well being which, in turn, benefits her children and her family.

66 *The first time I went out I felt wonderful — 15 minutes to the shop to get a take-away!* **99**

Mothers with a disability

There is no doubt that becoming a mother is a wonderful and exciting time, as you experience a range of intensity of emotions that you never imagined possible. It is a time of amazing change and growth and inevitably there will be some difficulties in making the necessary adjustments. To start with, things may seem very fraught until you become used to having a baby in your life and, as a mother with a disability, there may be extra factors which you need to consider.

You may have difficulties with balance and co-ordination, lifting and carrying the baby or washing and dressing her. If you have a visual or hearing impairment, you may be particularly anxious about safety considerations. The problems will vary according to the disability.

It is very difficult to provide specific information on all disabilities and how they may affect your life as a mother. The information in this chapter is intended to offer some general guidelines as well as sources of further information. It contains helpful suggestions from mothers with a disability, based on what they found useful themselves.

Most new mothers get extremely tired in the early months, partly due to the sleepless nights and partly due to the physical demands of pregnancy and birth. For mothers with a disability, the tiredness experienced is likely to be greater because of the lack of mobility and the increased physical demands created by your disability. It is all too easy to underestimate this tiredness and to blame it entirely on your disability. Do make allowances and ask for and accept all offers of help. Discuss with the people who are helping you what specific practical help will be the most useful to you.

Much of the extra stress you experience at this time, may be caused to a large extent by a lack of information or resources and the attitudes and actions of people you come into contact with. Recognising this and tackling it early on can be a useful way of reducing stress at this stage in your life.

You will probably already have had contact with a number of different health professionals and may well have developed a good relationship with the ones you meet regularly. Suddenly you find yourself in a new situation having to make new contacts and possibly feeling very vulnerable, insecure and lacking in confidence. This probably has nothing to do with your disability – these feelings are shared by the majority of new mothers.

Many health visitors or midwives will not have had any direct experience of caring for people with your particular disability. Rather than encouraging and allowing you to develop your confidence as a mother and working out your own strategies of caring for your family, they may seem overprotective and patronising. They may constantly be offering advice on what you should do. This may or may not be particuary helpful, depending on whether it takes into consideration any specific limitations caused by your disability.

Just remember that you know best what you can and can't manage, as you are used to coping with the day-to-day restrictions that your disability causes. If you can work closely with the health visitor and midwife, combining their expertise and experience of babycare with your knowledge and understanding of your own situation, together you should be able to work out how best to care for your baby.

You will also find the physiotherapist or occupational therapist can offer help and advice on how to modify equipment or the way you tackle certain jobs, such as lifting or bathing the baby. An organisation called REMAP has some 2,000 members, all volunteers among whom are engineers, technicians and craftsmen, physiotherapists and occupational therapists who can help in adapting existing equipment to your specific needs. All you need to pay for is the cost of materials (see Useful Addresses at the end of the book).

It may be difficult to work out exactly what you will need before the baby arrives – this is when talking to someone in a similar position is useful as they can suggest things they have found helpful. The more prepared you are before the baby arrives the better.

Many women find that the early days at home with a new baby are extremely lonely. They may know very few people in their neighbourhood if they have always gone out to work. If you are disabled you may experience this feeling of isolation even more acutely, as transporting yourself and a small baby may be difficult and access to many public places for people with a disability is still very limited in both towns and rural areas.

The NCT has branches all over the country and most of them run postnatal support schemes which provide both support and encouragement for new mums on a mother-to-mother basis. They will often provide transport for mothers who don't drive and may well come to some mutual arrangement about helping with the shopping or babyminding. Contact your local NCT branch to find out about their postnatal groups. You do not need to have attended NCT classes to take advantage of the other activities your local branch can offer.

Both the NCT and Maternity Alliance have a disabled mothers' working group which may be able to offer you helpful information, or put you in touch with another mother who has a similar disability. You may find it helpful to talk to someone who shares and understands your specific difficulties.

Before having a child, you may have thought that coffee mornings or mother and toddler groups, where mothers sit around talking endlessly about babies and nappies, would not be your scene. Most mothers benefit from talking to others who are experiencing or have just been through, a particular stage with their baby and you will probably find that developing those contacts will help reduce the feeling of loneliness.

LOOKING AFTER YOURSELF

The day-to-day routine tasks tend to take longer when you are disabled and inevitably that means you will find it hard to make time for yourself in the midst of juggling all the chores that need to be done.

It will be particularly important for you to work out your priorities and to decide what jobs could be left to another time.

You may need to change the way you do things at present. Use the time planning sheet on page 105 and look at things that you can do less often rather than on a daily basis. Experience will teach you how to take short cuts to reduce the time it takes to complete various tasks, but initially it is important to try and keep frustration to a minimum by not taking on too much all at once.

If you have a visual or hearing impairment, you are likely to suffer from a lot of muscle tension. When you are coping with unfamiliar surroundings or tackling unfamiliar tasks, there is a tendency to use more muscles of the body than you need as you are concentrating so hard on what you are doing. If joint stiffness or muscular weakness is a feature of your particular disability, then you are likely to feel tense and exhausted more quickly.

Allowing time for rest and relaxation in between activities may be better for you than pushing yourself and collapsing at the end of the day on the point of exhaustion.

Relaxation will allow you to feel refreshed and able to tackle things again with renewed energy. Try to set aside some time during each day to relax, you will find that it pays off in the long run.

Exercise also makes you healthier and can make you feel revitalised and relaxed, providing it is the right sort for you.

Any increase in activity levels is likely to be beneficial, especially if it is done instead of some boring routine and exhausting chore. The key is to sort out which boring routine chores can be dropped without feeling guilty about them.

Sharon and her husband are registered blind. They have a little boy called David who is eight-months-old. She relates her experience. "I spent 4 days in hospital and at first the nurses wouldn't let me do anything. Finally, I had to insist that they let me learn how to handle David myself. At first all I wanted to do was hold him all the time. I breastfed him for 2 weeks and then I put him onto the bottle.

"At first it was difficult finding out how we would mix his feeds as we couldn't see but our health visitor was able to get ready mixed baby milk feeds for us. We have large litre cartons for day-to-day feeds and I use talking scales to fill the bottles. We have little cartons with 250 ml (8 fl oz) in for travelling. A number of the most popular brands of baby milk are available in this form.

"I was surprised at how quickly we settled into a routine at home. I had had a dummy run before I had him, thinking out where I would change him and where he would sleep for example.

"Now that he is older, I sometimes use a playpen, although I don't like to restrict him to it all the time. I can hear where he is and we have made sure that the room is safe. Once he is mobile, things will be a bit more difficult.

"My health visitor gave us a syringe for giving David medicine for sore throats or teething. It holds exactly the right amount of liquid as accurate measuring would be difficult for us.

"My main advice to other blind mothers would be never give up because of your eyesight. Persevere and find a way around a problem."

A mother with multiple sclerosis who has a seven-and-a-half-month-old daughter talks of her experiences of motherhood.

"The most helpful thing was knowing that others had got through it. I was a career girl and having to give up my job soon after I became pregnant because the travelling got too much, was very hard. Once I had the baby, I really enjoyed being at home with her after all those hard months of being at home alone.

"I have difficulty in walking and standing. Around the house I have a number of different stools placed in appropriate places so that I can sit down to do most things. When we go out, I use a wheelchair and so I always need someone else to push the chair while I hold the baby on my lap. I used a sling initially and now she is a bit older I use a harness to keep her from falling.

"I had an easy labour but had to stay in hospital for 7 days to fit in with my husband's job so that he could have more time off work when I came home. I hated it in hospital as I had so much conflicting advice. Being at home was much better.

"We have the nursery downstairs so that once I am downstairs in the mornings everything I need during the day is within easy reach.

"When she was three months old I had a relapse and had to have steroids. I got terribly depressed for a while and then all of a sudden things got better again. She slept through the night at 5 weeks which has been a big help. I think I would be much more tired otherwise.

"My husband has been wonderful and he has been surprised at how much he enjoys being a dad. Being an only child with only one cousin, he hadn't had much contact with small babies before."

Sue is a mother with cerebral palsy, which affects her muscle control and co-ordination, resulting in irregular and jerky movements. She explains how she copes with her eight-month-old son Mark.

"I found it difficult at first coping with the demands of being a mother when all through my working life I had tended to avoid situations that were difficult for me. Now I had to find a way of managing.

> **❝I have had to re-organise when and how I get the shopping done, for example, to fit round the baby because I can't carry him and the shopping.❞**

"I tried to organise as much as possible before Mark was born. As I have difficulty with fine finger movements, I got my home help to sew velcro fasteners in place of poppers on all the babygros. We arranged for someone to come and fit a folding changing table onto the wall in the downstairs toilet. It has a large wooden clasp to hold it in place and easily folds down above the toilet at the correct height for me to stand and change Mark's nappy. It is very convenient as the wash basin and toilet are right there.

"I have fixed loops of tape through the clips on the cot so that I can manage to secure and release the cot sides more easily. Similar loops of tape are threaded through the ends of the zip fasteners on my feeding bras so that I can easily hook one finger into the loop and unzip the bra for feeding.

"I find it hard to clip and unclip the hooks on child harnesses, so the answer is to have a number of different sets, one on the high chair, one on the pushchair. It is very important to try out prams and pushchairs before you buy one as they vary so much.

"In the bath, I use a small reclining frame that looks like a smaller version of the bouncing chair. It has a detachable towelling cover which supports the baby in a reclining position that keeps his head well out of the water and gives me a free hand as I don't have to hold him in position. It is called a Batheasy Baby support. I have the baby bath on the table right next to a changing surface in Mark's bedroom. The bath has a plug hole in it which makes emptying it into a bucket underneath much easier than trying to carry it full of water.

"It is useful to have more than one set of spoons now that Mark is helping to feed himself, as he keeps throwing them on the floor, which is a great game for him but not so easy for me to keep bending down to pick them up.

"I use a small hand-held food processor to purée his food, which I find very useful.

"When carrying Mark downstairs, I hold him close to me and sit down and bump down each step on my bottom. I feel this is much safer for both of us. My home help comes with us when we go out shopping.

"I have enjoyed being a mother so much and have a wonderful little boy. When my disability causes a problem, I just have to find another way of doing the task. If I can't, I have to accept help from someone else. You just have to accept that there are some things that you won't be able to do."

• • • • • •

Sensible eating and weight control

There is probably no such thing as the 'ideal weight' a woman should gain in pregnancy, but there is a lot of debate and argument. Most women gain about 12.5 kg (2 stone).

You may have talked to some women who were not given any advice about how much weight they should gain and others who were monitored and told off for gaining too much. Whatever your weight gain was, it is important to realise that it will take time to return to normal weight, so try not to be disheartened.

Your weight gain is due mainly to the increasing size of the baby, the placenta, uterus, amniotic fluid, extra blood and the fat stores your body set aside. As soon as the baby is born you will lose some of that weight. The baby will probably weigh 2.7–4 kg (6–9 lb) and the placenta and fluid will probably account for another 900 g–1.3 kg (2–3 lb). Over the next few days you may lose 900 g–1.3 kg (2–3 lb) as your body gets rid of extra fluid and blood that is no longer needed. The uterus takes about 6 weeks to shrink from its pregnant size of approximately 900 g (2 lb) to its normal size of 50–75 g (2–3 oz). The remainder of the weight is likely to be made up of fat stores, some of which will be used up when you produce breastmilk for your baby.

During the early months of breastfeeding, you will probably find that you are more hungry and thirsty than usual. You should drink as and when you feel thirsty – it is a good idea to have a drink beside you when you sit down to feed. Water is perfectly adequate; you do not need to drink milk to make milk. If you like milk try not to drink too much of it as it is very high in fat and calories unless it is skimmed milk. You will need an extra 600 calories a day to ensure an adequate supply of breastmilk. A wholemeal sandwich, a slice of fruit cake and two pieces of fruit would equal about 600 calories.

You should not need to eat a special diet when breastfeeding, although you do need to make sure you are getting enough calcium and iron. Following the sensible guidelines below will ensure an adequate intake of nutrients for you and your baby. You may well come across all sorts of advice about what not to eat, like chocolate, strawberries, onions and so on, if you are breastfeeding. All babies are individuals and what one baby will tolerate quite happily another may react strongly against. Babies in India cope very well with curry while those in Mexico don't seem at all bothered by hot chillies.

If you think something you have eaten has disagreed with your baby, leave it off the menu for a few days and then try again. If it has the same reaction then you may have to refrain from eating that particular food until the baby is older and her digestive system more mature, or until she has been weaned off the breast. Some women suspect that cows milk in their own diet affects their baby and causes colic. If you are concerned, do discuss this with your health visitor or breastfeeding counsellor. A cows milk-free diet sheet is available from the breastfeeding promotion group (BPG) office at NCT HQ. Send a stamped addressed envelope.

You may feel very disheartened by the flabby state of your muscles and the excess weight which you may find hard to get rid of but try not to think about actually 'dieting' especially if you are breastfeeding. Being at least 3.1 kg (half a stone) overweight at the end of pregnancy is very common. This seems to be the body's way of providing a fat reserve for the lactation period and it is thought that prolactin, the hormone responsble for milk production has a tendency to retain fluid. Following sensible eating and exercise guidelines will probably mean that you lose weight gradually over the months you breastfeed, or that you maintain your present weight until you finish breastfeeding when you will probably find that the extra weight drops off. If it does not, that will be the time to work harder at losing the excess weight.

Being very overweight does cause certain problems such as excess strain and wear and tear on joints like the knees, hips and back and also means more strain for your heart which has to pump blood to all body cells including the fat cells. Also, your chances of having high blood pressure are increased if you are very overweight. So it is important that you do try to eventually reach an ideal weight for your height but remember, it took nine months for the weight to be gained, so don't expect to lose it overnight. If you were overweight before you became pregnant, then you should make allowances for that too.

Check your weight against the chart below and see which band you fall into. Remember

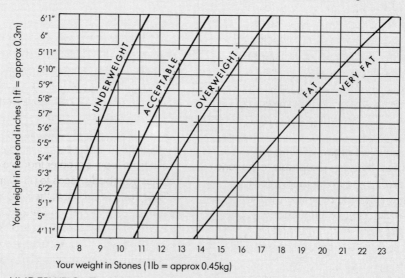

The chart shown below was produced by the Health Education Authority. It gives the acceptable weight ranges for men and women which carry the least health risk. Draw a horizontal line across the chart for your height.

UNDERWEIGHT – Are you eating enough?
ACCEPTABLE – This is the desirable weight range for health.
OVERWEIGHT – Not likely to affect your health but don't get any fatter.
FAT – Your health could suffer if you don't loose weight.
VERY FAT – This is severe and treatment is urgently required.

when you read the chart that you have just had a baby so don't be too disheartened if you are into the next band. It will give you some idea of the target weight to aim for which will be right for your height. Be specific about how much weight you want to lose and then be realistic and allow yourself time to reach that target. People who take time to lose weight gradually rather than those who aim for a sudden dramatic weight loss are usually able to maintain that weight loss.

To lose weight effectively, safely and permanently requires alterations on both eating and exercise patterns.

It has been shown that going on a drastic diet is not the most efficient way to lose weight. A very low calorie diet may lead you to lose a lot of weight initially but it can often be fluid and muscle protein that is being lost rather than stored body fat. This type of diet is likely to be difficult to maintain for any length of time. Boredom with the diet, lack of energy and general lethargy set in and it's all too easy to abandon the diet and revert to all the bad eating habits again.

Small, gradual changes in eating and exercise patterns that are acceptable to you and your family are likely to be far more effective and are the sort that you can stick to in the future. In the early days of motherhood, you won't want to be bothered with carefully watching everything you eat and counting all your calories.

The ideal diet should be easy to prepare and fit in with normal daily routine. It should contain enough calories so that you are not feeling constantly fatigued and enable you to maintain your target weight. It should not require any drastic changes to your social habits and should contain a wide variety of different foods.

66After 4 months people expect you to be back to normal. For the first few weeks everyone says how well you look — but at 4 months going swimming!!!99

A lot of people think of food in terms of good and bad foods and then eat as much as they can manage of the so called good ones and spend the rest of their time desperately trying to avoid the bad ones. Rather than following this principle, it is much better to look at the overall balance of your diet. Provided you follow some basic guidelines, you should be able to make your own choices about the food you eat. A cream cake or a bar of chocolate is not the end of the world as long as you don't eat them all the time. It is the overall balance of your diet that matters.

THE BALANCE BETWEEN CALORIES IN AND OUT

The different foods that you eat, such as proteins, carbohydrates or fats, all contain variable amounts of energy. Your body requires energy for all the different functions it has to perform daily, such as breathing and keeping your heart beating, blinking your eyes, walking, talking, sleeping and so on. The energy stored in food and the energy used by the muscles for work is measured in calories. If your calorie intake from food is greater than the amount of calories your body needs to perform everyday activities and repair itself, then the extra unused calories are converted and stored in your body as body fat. If you consistently eat 50 calories a day more than you need, those extra calories will be stored as body fat and that is likely to be about 3.1 kg (half a stone) a year. It is all a question of the balance between calories TAKEN IN and calories BURNT UP which is important in weight control.

• • • • • •

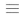
WHAT IS A GOOD HEALTHY DIET?

In the past people spent a large proportion of the day working on the land and in factories. At times there were shortages of food and a balanced diet of three square meals a day with meat and two vegetables and plenty of protein and dairy produce was considered important to ensure that everyone had enough of the correct nutrients. Lifestyles have changed considerably in the past 100 years. The problems facing us nowadays are likely to be a lack of activity and exercise and an overabundance of food, especially food derived from animals and highly processed foods which tend to be high in fat and sugar.

In 1983 the government set up a committee, the National Advisory Committee on Nutritional Education, to look at the nation's eating patterns and produce some recommendations. Their report which became known as the NACNE report recommended that we should change our diets to reduce our intake of fat, sugar and salt, and increase our intake of fibre.

INGREDIENTS FOR HEALTHY EATING

There is such a wide variety of natural ingredients to choose from for a healthy diet, that eating well will always be interesting and exciting.

Meat is an excellent source of first class protein, which means that it does not have to be combined with other ingredients in order to give you the right type of protein your body needs.

Fish and shellfish are also a superb source of high-quality protein.

Fresh vegetables play a large part in a healthy diet. The different types provide a wide variety of vitamins and minerals and all provide significant amounts of dietary fibre.

Fruits provide a healthy and natural sweetness. They are an excellent source of dietary fibre and none contain more than a trace of fat.

Pulses are an important source of protein, particularly in a vegetarian diet, but they must be eaten with grain products to provide the best protein.

Nuts and seeds, when mixed with whole grain ingredients, will provide a high protein meal.

All grains provide protein and, when mixed with other second class protein ingredients such as nuts or pulses, will provide good quality protein for healthy growth and repair of body tissue.

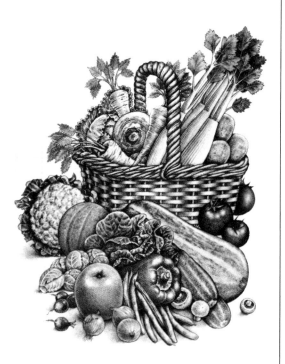

HEALTHY EATING QUIZ

The quiz below is to help you analyse your present eating patterns and to indicate where changes may be necessary. Answer each question carefully and choose the most appropriate answer i.e. never, occasionally, frequently, daily, putting the corresponding number of points in the last column. Add up the totals and check below for the results.

ANSWERS		
NEVER	1	
OCCASIONALLY (once a week or less)	2	
FREQUENTLY (three or more times/week)	3	
DAILY	4	
How often do you eat the following?		
SECTION A		
Wholemeal bread		
Brown rice or wholemeal pasta		
Vegetables		
Fruit		
Fish (not fried)		
Cottage cheese		
Skimmed or semi-skimmed milk		
Low fat spread		
Muesli, porridge or high fibre cereal		
Chicken or turkey		
TOTAL		

SECTION B	
White bread	
White rice or ordinary pasta	
Ice cream	
Fried foods	
Full fat milk	
Full fat or hard cheese	
Offal (kidney, liver etc.)	
Eggs	
Chips	
Processed breakfast cereals, such as cornflakes	
Butter or hard margarine	
Sausages	
Burgers	
Pies	
Cakes and biscuits	
TOTAL	

ANSWERS: Add up your totals for the two sections. If your points total for section A is higher than section B, then you have a fairly good diet already, with a fair proportion of fibre and not too much fat. If the total for section B is much higher than section A, then you need to look at where you can make some changes to your eating habits in order to reduce the points for section B and increase those for section A.

• • • • • •   • • • • • •

FAT: WHY DO WE NEED IT?

Certain important fat-soluble vitamins are found in foods that contain fat. These are vitamins A, D, E and K. As the body is able to store these vitamins, it is not essential to have a source of these every day. (See pages 128 and 129 for information about which foods contain which vitamins and why they are needed.)

Fat also provides energy for the body's requirements but the energy from fat is a very concentrated source. Every gram of fat in your diet will produce 9 Calories of energy, which is twice what a gram of carbohydrates will produce. This is why it is so easy to consume many more calories than we need if we have a lot of fat in the diet. However, some fat stores are necessary in the body both to provide protection for our internal organs and also for insulation – helping to prevent excessive heat loss from the body when it is exposed to very low temperatures.

WHAT IS FAT?

You will have seen food labels marked 'high in polyunsaturates', 'low in saturates' 'low in cholesterol', but what does all this mean? It can all be very confusing.

Fats are made up of substances called fatty acids, which are chains of carbon and hydrogen atoms linked together. Depending on the way in which the atoms of hydrogen and carbon are combined together, they are divided into the two main groups – saturated and unsaturated fats. Because of their different chemical structures, they have different effects on the body.

Saturated fats are linked with raised cholesterol levels in the blood which can lead to an increased risk of coronary heart disease. Unsaturated fats can be divided into two groups: monounsaturated fats and polyunsaturated fats. Polyunsaturated fats may actually lower the level of cholesterol in the blood.

Most foods contain a mixture of saturated and unsaturated fatty acids, but are mainly one type or the other. What is important, is to know which foods contain saturated fats and which contain unsaturated fats, so you can reduce your overall fat intake, especially saturated fat.

Saturated fats tend to be hard at room temperature. They are found mainly in animal fats such as meat (pork, beef and lamb), lard, dripping, suet, dairy products such as milk, cream and cheese, chocolate, hard margarines, palm and coconut oil present in biscuits and cakes, sauces and puddings. Processed foods often contain fats which are listed as hydrogenated vegetable fat/oils. Hydrogenated oils are also saturated – they have been saturated with hydrogen to make them hard.

Vegetable oils are generally unsaturated fats, with the exceptions of coconut and palm oil which, although of vegetable origin, are saturated fats because of their chemical composition. Manufactured cakes and biscuits often use these types of oil, so it is always wise to look at the labels. Buying a bottle of blended vegetable oil means that you don't always know which types of vegetable oils have gone into the product. They may contain saturated fats, so it is usually advisable to choose an oil which clearly states that it is high in monounsaturates, such as olive oil, or polyunsaturates, such as sunflower or safflower oil.

Monounsaturated fats are found mainly in olive oil and peanut oil.

Polyunsaturated fats are found mainly in vegetable oils, like sunflower, corn and soya oils, nuts and oily fish like herrings, mackerel and trout, and soft spreads labelled high in polyunsaturates.

There is a lot of confusion about

margarines and spreads. All butter and margarines must by law contain 82% fat. Anything with less fat in it must be called a spread. Some spreads have between 60% and 75% fat while others have lower amounts. Their weight is made up with water. It is important to read the labels carefully looking at the overall fat content and the amounts of saturated and unsaturated fats so you can compare the products and choose the most appropriate one.

The modern health message is that we should reduce the total amount of fat that we eat, especially saturated fat. This can be done by reducing the overall amount of fat we consume as well as using polyunsaturated fats in place of saturated fat whenever possible. A high fat intake is more likely to lead to an increase in blood pressure and to being overweight. Too much saturated fat is likely to lead to an increase in blood cholesterol levels and as there is some evidence that this is linked with a higher risk of coronary heart disease, it would be sensible to reduce our intake.

WHAT IS CHOLESTEROL?

Cholesterol is a white fat-like substance which is manufactured in the liver. It is essential for the normal function of cell membranes and in the production of hormones and bile (which is necessary for digesting food). Our bodies manufacture cholesterol from the animal fat in our diets.

Consuming more saturated fat than we need can result in raised levels of cholesterol circulating in the blood stream. There is some evidence to suggest that this may cause an increase in the fatty deposits which stick to the walls of the arteries and cause narrowing. This condition, known as arteriosclerosis, is a contributing factor in coronary heart disease. When the arteries are too narrow, the blood

supply to a part of the heart or brain may be blocked off, and this results in a heart attack or stroke.

You may think this is only likely to happen to older people, but furring up of the arteries has been found in surprisingly young adults and teenagers.

In some families with a history of heart disease, there may be an inherited tendency to high cholesterol levels. For those families, it may be helpful to ask for a cholesterol test to check what theirs is. Reducing the amount of animal fats you consume can lower cholesterol levels, which will greatly reduce the risks of heart disease.

Egg yolks, shellfish and offal are particularly rich in cholesterol and should be eaten in moderation only. Plants cannot manufacture cholesterol so there is none in vegetables and fruit. There is some evidence that eating a high fibre diet helps to reduce cholesterol levels.

HOW TO EAT LESS FAT

When trying to cut down on your fat intake, look at the list of suggestions below and choose the ones that might be easiest for you to change – don't try and make all the changes at once. Try one first and then gradually add in others week by week. If you make the changes little by little, you are more likely to stick to them.

● Change from full cream milk (silver top) to semi-skimmed or skimmed milk. It may take a little while to adjust your taste buds but persevere and eventually you will find it hard to go back to drinking the full cream type. Both have just as much calcium as full cream milk but far less fat. However, skimmed milk is not recommended for children under five.

Fat content of milk:

1 pint silver top	22 grams
1 pint semi-skimmed milk	11 grams
1 pint skimmed	1 gram

- When buying meat, choose the leanest cut you can afford. Cut off all visible fat.
- Substitute chicken, turkey and fish for meat a few times a week. Remove all skin from the poultry as this is where a lot of the fat is stored.
- Use a non-stick pan as this means you can use much less oil (you may not need any at all). When roasting meat in the oven, stand it on a rack to allow any fat to drain off the meat during cooking.
- Try a vegetarian meal without meat occasionally – you may even find you prefer it. Try substituting pulses, such as chickpeas or lentils for meat.
- Choose a low fat spread rather than butter or margarine and spread it thinly. Do without the spread if you are using a topping.
- Cut down on crisps, cakes, chocolates, pies and pastry.
- If you like cheese, remember that the hard and cream cheeses tend to have the highest fat content; Edam and Brie are medium fat and cottage cheese has the lowest fat content of all the cheeses.
- Choose low fat yoghurt instead of cream sometimes. If you must use cream, use single instead of double.
- Use Quark (soft cheese) which is low in fat and can be used in cooking instead of full fat soft cheese.
- Grill rather than fry your food.
- Grill or steam fish rather than frying in a batter which will absorb a lot of fat.
- When using cooking oil or fat, use as little as possible and choose one that is low in saturated fats.
- Try stir frying using a steep-sided, round-bottomed pan like a wok as this allows you to use very little oil.
- Thick straight cut chips are better than thin or crinkly ones which will absorb more fat. Use a sunflower, soya or corn oil for frying. Alternatively, try oven chips. Try not to have chips too often.

SUGAR: WHY DO WE NEED IT?

Well actually we don't! Sugar is a type of carbohydrate which provides energy in the form of calories but provides no nutrients whatsoever.

We need energy (calories) for all our daily activities but we also need other nutrients for the normal growth and functioning of our bodies. If we eat a lot of foods high in sugar, which don't provide any other nutrients, rather than a well-balanced diet, we may be lacking in certain nutrients that are essential for good health.

Sugary foods, while high in calories don't contain fibre and therefore don't help to fill us up, making it easy to eat too much – i.e. more calories than our body will burn up with the result that the surplus is stored as fat. Unfortunately, our taste buds have a tendency to crave sweet things which makes it easy to eat more.

Eating sugar also increases the risk of tooth decay. How often we eat sugar, tends to be more important than how much is eaten. The bacteria in the mouth feed on the sugar and produce acid which attacks teeth. If endless sugary snacks are eaten, the teeth are constantly bathed in a sugary solution and never have a chance to recover.

You may say when asked, 'I don't take sugar' thinking mainly of the common form of white or brown sugar you buy in shops. This is found naturally in sugar cane and sugar beet and is known as sucrose. It is processed to produce sugar as we know it.

However, there are various other types of sugar which are used in all sorts of manufactured products. These sugars are known as dextrose, glucose, glucose syrup, fructose, lactose, maltose etc. All these sugars are the same in terms of nutrition; they contain no vitamins, minerals or protein.

• • • • • •

HOW TO EAT LESS SUGAR

- Choose fruit juice or low-calorie drinks instead of ordinary soft drinks. There are the equivalent of 5 teaspoons of sugar in a can of cola.
- Choose canned fruit in natural juice rather than in syrup.
- Look at the labels on everything you buy. You will soon get to know which brands to choose. Ingredients have to be listed in order of the amount included.
- Don't add sugar to baby foods or drinks. It will only encourage a sweet tooth.
- Try not to use sweets as a reward.
- Cakes and biscuits tend to have a lot of sugar in them, so cut down on these.
- You can usually reduce (halve in some cases) the amount of sugar in most recipes, apart from meringues and jam, without having any adverse effects on the results.
- Try having fresh fruit instead of sweet puddings at some meals.
- Foods with a naturally occurring sugar content, like dried fruit, can be used to sweeten food.
- Try not to eat foods containing sugar in between meals.

SALT: WHY DO WE NEED IT?

Salt is a natural substance which consists of sodium and chloride, both of which are necessary elements for the body. Sodium is needed for the normal functioning of nerves and muscles while chloride is important in digestion. Salt is used in food as a preservative and to enhance flavour.

In Britain we eat about 10 grams of salt a day. About half of that amount comes from salt added to manufactured food, the other half is added in cooking, or at the table or occurs naturally in food. We only NEED about one gram a day.

Too much salt can lead to high blood pressure in some people, which can contribute to heart disease and strokes. It is difficult to predict which people might be more susceptible to these conditions, so it is sensible for everyone to try and cut down on salt.

Salt attracts fluid and a high salt intake may contribute to any tendency to retain fluid. Some women suffer from this tendency just before their periods and cutting down on salt can help to reduce this.

Young babies find it difficult to deal with salt; they should not have any added to food.

HOW TO EAT LESS SALT

Have a good variety of foods in your diet, so that you get all the salt you need without adding any extra. In addition, look at the list below and decide which one you might be able to do, then gradually make the other changes that are acceptable, little by little.

- Try using very little salt in cooking and use flavourings like herbs and spices instead.
- Many people add salt to food at the table without even tasting it first. Don't put the salt on the table and that should reduce the tendency to add salt to everything.

- If you buy canned vegetables look at the label and choose ones with no added salt.
- Try making your own home-made soup rather than always relying on packet and canned soups which tend to have quite a lot of salt added.
- Crisps and salted peanuts can add a lot of salt in your diet. Try to cut down on these.
- Gammon and bacon both have high salt concentrations, so eat these in moderation.

By cutting down on your salt intake you will probably find that you get used to the taste of food without salt. If you really miss salt you could try using low salt substitutes, but these tend to be high in potassium and while this may not cause any problems for the majority of people there are some for whom too much potassium could be harmful, small babies and those with kidney problems in particular. Using salt (and sugar) substitutes may seem useful in the short term but it would be healthier if you could reduce your taste for salt and sugar.

FIBRE: WHY DO WE NEED IT?

Fibre is essential to the normal functioning of the intestines. Many of the diseases prevalent in the Western World, like digestive disorders and coronary heart disease, are thought to be related to a lack of fibre, or roughage, in our diet. These diseases are far less common in the third world although they are found amongst people who emigrate to the West and adopt Western-style diets.

Fibre is the name given to a special group of carbohydrates. Fibre forms the skeleton of plants. It is found in the outer covering of many grains, fruits and vegetables; it is often removed in modern processing methods.

Fibre is not digested as it passes through the digestive system and so doesn't provide any nutrients itself, but the foods that are naturally high in fibre are a good source of vitamins and other nutrients.

Instead, fibre helps food to pass through the intestines more quickly, which can minimise the absorption of various harmful substances and makes conditions such as bowel cancer less likely.

Piles (or haemorrhoids) and constipation are prevented by an adequate intake of fibre because it absorbs water and helps to make the stools soft and bulky so that they can be eliminated without straining.

Diverticulitis which is now the commonest disease of the large intestine in the West, was very rare in the early part of this century in the West and is hardly known at all in the rural districts of Africa and Asia where the people consume about two and a half times more fibre than we do in the West.

Foods with a high fibre content are satisfying and fill you up without giving you too many calories. For instance, 550 g (1¼ lb) of potatoes contain the same number of calories as 100 g (4 oz) of cheese (about 460 calories).

There are two main types of fibre, soluble and insoluble. Soluble fibre dissolves in water, hence the name. It is found mainly in cereals – especially oats, vegetables – especially beans, and some fruits. Insoluble fibre absorbs and holds onto water, so is responsible for making soft bulky stools and helping to move the food through the intestines quickly. It is found in cereals like wheat and bran and vegetables.

It is important to eat both types of fibre, but all you need to do is ensure that you have a variety of different fibre-rich foods. It is better to get your fibre from foods rather than supplements which you add to the diet like bran. Most Britains consume about 20 grams of fibre a day but the recommended amount is 30 grams a day.

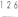

SOURCES OF FIBRE

Good sources of fibre are breakfast cereals, leafy and root vegetables, fruits – fresh and dried, bread, rice, pasta and nuts.

The following table shows you approximate fibre content of some common foods to give you an idea of just how much fibre 30 grams is. It is best to increase your intake gradually over a number of weeks as a sudden change to high fibre foods can cause unpleasant wind or an uncomfortable bloated feeling.

WAYS TO INCREASE FIBRE

- Eat more fruit and vegetables
- Eat more potatoes especially with their jackets on
- Used canned or dried beans
- Eat more nuts (unsalted) and dried fruit
- Use wholemeal flour instead of white flour or try half and half
- Eat more wholemeal bread
- Try to use high fibre breakfast cereals.

FIBRE CONTENT OF SOME COMMON FOODS

VEGETABLES AND BEANS (1 serving)		
Peas	7	grams
Sweetcorn	5	grams
Carrots	3	grams
Baked beans	6	grams
Red kidney beans	10	grams
Tomatoes	1.2	grams
Jacket potatoes	3	grams
FRUIT		
1 Banana	3	grams
1 Apple	2	grams
1 Grapefruit	0.6	grams
30g (1oz) Raisins	2	grams
2 dried apricots	7	grams
BREAD (4 slices)		
Wholemeal bread	11	grams
White bread	3	grams
Brown bread	6	grams

RICE (1 serving)		
Brown	3	grams
White	2	grams
SPAGHETTI (1 serving)		
Ordinary	2	grams
Wholemeal	6	grams
BREAKFAST CEREALS (1 serving)		
Puffed wheat	4	grams
Porridge	3	grams
Weetabix (2)	5	grams
Cornflakes	2	grams
All bran	10	grams
NUTS (1 tablespoon)		
Brazils	2.3	grams
Almonds	3.6	grams
Peanuts, roasted	2	grams

Figures quoted in different publications may vary slightly depending on which method of measuring the fibre content has been used.

VITAMINS AND MINERALS

Vitamins and minerals are vital to the healthy functioning of the body and a deficiency in certain vitamins and minerals can lead to disease. In the West with the wide variety of foods available, it is highly unlikely that anyone would suffer from any deficiency. Most people eating a variety of foods do not need to add vitamin or mineral supplements to their diets.

You may have been advised during your pregnancy to take iron and folic acid supplements. However, there is evidence which shows that there is no real clinical benefit to be gained either in the pregnancy or by the baby. The mother's iron stores may be improved but there is no evidence to suggest that all pregnant women benefit from iron and folic acid supplements. Blood tests will show those women whose haemoglobin levels are low and they should be treated accordingly.

WHY ARE VITAMINS AND MINERALS IMPORTANT

VITAMIN A (retinol) is essential for good vision, healthy skin and strong bones and also for resistance to infection.

VITAMIN B_1 (thiamin) helps the body to use the carbohydrates to provide energy. It is also needed for growth and for healthy muscles and nerves.

VITAMIN B_2 (riboflavin) helps the body to produce energy from fat, protein and carbohydrates. It is also needed for healthy tissues, especially skin and eyes.

VITAMIN B_3 (niacin) helps healthy functioning of skin, nerves and digestive system.

VITAMIN B_6 (pyridoxine) is needed for the formation of red blood cells and is necessary for brain function.

VITAMIN B_{12} (cobalamin) is needed for growth and the formation of blood cells.

FOLIC ACID (folate) is needed for the formation of red blood cells, cell formation and cell immunity to disease.

VITAMIN C (ascorbic acid) is important for energy production and growth, healthy gums, skin and bones and resistance to infection and wound healing.

VITAMIN D is essential for the efficient absorption of calcium from the diet and is necessary for healthy bones and teeth.

VITAMIN E protects vitamins A and C from being destroyed by acting as an antioxidant and also helping the body use vitamin K.

VITAMIN K is important for blood clotting.

CALCIUM is important for healthy bones and teeth, heartbeat, blood clotting and muscle contractions.

IRON is needed for healthy tissues and blood.

PHOSPHORUS is needed with calcium for strong bones and teeth. It is necessary for the release of energy from food and is a vital component of body cells. Phosphorus is important for muscle function.

SODIUM maintains the correct water balance of the body. It is also needed for muscles and nerves to function.

POTASSIUM helps regulate the heartbeat and normal muscle function and acts like sodium to control water balance.

There are many other minerals, such as zinc, magnesium, selenium, copper, iodine and fluoride, which are known as trace elements and are only needed by the body in very small amounts.

WHERE TO FIND THESE VITAMINS AND MINERALS

Wholemeal bread: Vitamins B_1, B_2, B_3, B_6, zinc, phosphorus, iron, magnesium and potassium.

Wholegrain cereals: B_1, B_2, B_3, B_6, E, phosphorus, iron, sodium, potassium, zinc, magnesium, selenium, copper and manganese.

Nuts: B_1, B_2, E, B_6, zinc, magnesium, copper and manganese.

Milk: B_1, B_2, B_6, B_{12}, D, K, calcium, phosphorus, potassium, zinc and magnesium.

Dairy products: A, B_2, B_3, D, calcium, phosphorus, sodium, zinc.

Fruit and vegetables:
Carrots: A.
Spinach: K, iron.
Broccoli: A, K, calcium, iron.
Leafy green vegetables: E, B_6, folic acid.
Dark green vegetables: C, B.
Peas: folic acid, magnesium and manganese.
Potatoes: C
Tomatoes: C
Dried beans: B_1, B_3, folic acid.
Vegetable oils: E.
Bananas: B_6, potassium, folic acid, magnesium.
Oranges: potassium, C, folic acid.
Dried apricots: A, iron, magnesium.
Citrus fruits, melons: C.

Meat: B_3, B_6, iron phosphorus.
Liver: A, D, B_1, B_2, B_3, B_6, B_{12}, K, folic acid, zinc and copper.

Eggs: A, D, B_3, B_{12}, iron, manganese, phosphorus.

Fish: A, D, B_2, B_3, B_6, B_{12}, calcium (sardines, salmon with bones), sodium, phosphorus.

It is important to remember that you may be lacking in iron following the birth of your baby, so do try to make sure that your diet contains the foods that are rich in iron. Vitamin C helps the body to absorb iron, so make sure you have plenty of foods rich in Vitamin C in your diet. Broccoli, peas, spinach, egg yolks, red meat and liver are all rich sources of iron.

Calcium is an important mineral to ensure adequate bone density. Women who have reached the menopause are at risk of osteoporosis (loss of bone density) due to the hormonal changes. This increases the chances of fracturing bones if you fall. If bone density is developed and maintained at a very good level from a young age, any loss after the menopause is likely to be less severe. It is better to eat and exercise at the correct level from childhood onwards rather than cramming in the supplements in middle age. Weight bearing exercise is another important factor in ensuring healthy bones.

Sardines, salmon or pilchards with bones, cottage cheese, low fat yoghurt, milk, spring greens and soya beans are all good sources of calcium. Substances found in alcohol, plant foods, whole grains and red meat tend to inhibit calcium absorption which is why a diet which contains a wide variety of foods rather than a high proportion of any one type is far more beneficial.

Vitamins and minerals are lost both in the storing and cooking of foods. Air, heat and sunlight all contribute to the loss of vitamins and minerals. To preserve the maximum amounts available in the food, you need to handle it carefully.

- Always buy the freshest possible produce.
- Store fresh vegetables in a cool dark place.
- Keep milk in a cool dark place.
- Use as little water as possible when cooking vegetables and cook them for the shortest possible time.
- Don't leave cooked food standing for too long before serving.
- Use the vegetable water to make stocks and gravy.

Too much of a particular vitamin or mineral can be dangerous. It is very rare to take too much in a normal diet, but it is possible to have an overdose if you take vitamins in supplements. Do follow the instructions about dose very carefully. Most people eating a good mixed diet do not need vitamin or mineral supplements. Vegetarians may be at risk of iron and vitamin B deficiency, so they should ensure that they have sufficient of the foods that include them.

You may worry about whether your baby or young child is getting enough vitamins and minerals in her diet. The Department of Health recommends that children under five should be given vitamin drops, but talk to your health visitor or doctor if you have any queries. Do make sure you follow the instructions about dosage carefully.

CHANGES IN EATING PATTERNS

Having looked at the information above, you may decide that you are already eating a fairly healthy diet or you may feel that you are going to need to make a lot of changes in order to be healthy. It may help to look at the many factors influencing why you eat in the way you do, such as upbringing, tradition, food availability, cost, social customs and pressures, advertising etc. This might help you make a start on altering your eating habits .

Many people admit that they rarely eat because they are hungry – they have been educated to eat at certain times of the day and to think of certain foods as being essential. This idea is not in keeping with current lifestyle and today's information about healthy eating. Often people eat more than they need because of a built-in notion that they should always eat up everything on their plate, which probably comes from childhood. As a mother yourself now, this is worth bearing in mind when your child gets to the stage of eating solids.

All children are individuals from the start and one baby will have a different feeding pattern from the next. In the early weeks and months when you are breastfeeding, it is better to feed on demand when the baby is hungry. This is by far the best way of ensuring a good milk supply and a contented and well-fed baby. If you are bottle feeding, it is also advisable to be reasonably flexible about feed times rather than rigidly clock watching. When the time comes to wean her onto solid food, you will probably want her to fit into the normal family patterns of eating but do remember that she may not always be hungry when you decide its lunchtime, so be prepared to be flexible about it.

Allow her to feed herself as soon as possible. It will be very messy to start with but it should encourage her to eat well and teach her new skills.

Many mothers with a small child are very anxious about whether or not their child is getting enough of the right nutrients and life can become very fraught at meal times. It may be hard to accept that your child has likes and dislikes about foods which you consider to be important. It helps to look at things from your child's perspective.

It must be quite daunting to be faced with a huge plateful of food you don't like when you're not feeling very hungry, especially if you know from experience that the person you love will be angry if you don't eat everything on the plate.

Try to keep calm and not lose your temper if your child rejects something you have lovingly prepared for him or her. It is easy to underestimate the effects your anger might be having. One child said 'Don't be cross with me, please, mummy. It makes me feel so lonely.'

Follow the handy hints given below and you should be able to avoid mealtime tantrums.

- Give your child some choice in the matter of what he eats.
- Put a number of different foods on the table and let him help himself.
- Sandwiches are very nutritious, especially when made with wholemeal bread. Suggest a number of different fillings and let him choose the one he wants.
- Allow him to decide when he's had enough, while making sure that he doesn't just say that he's full, because he knows there is a sweet treat coming up later. If you offer fruit or yoghurt as a second course you might avoid this problem.
- Small children hardly ever starve themselves provided they are offered a variety of foods. They may go through a phase when all they will eat is fish fingers and bananas but remember that they are probably still getting a lot of nutrients from milk. Try not to get too anxious about food or you could make the problem worse.
- Don't waste time cooking elaborate meals for your toddler in the middle of the day. Simple foods like baked beans, fish fingers, bread and cheese and fruit or yoghurt are all nourishing and easy to prepare, and you won't feel you have wasted a lot of time if he doesn't eat it all.
- Avoid too many snacks in between meals as they will spoil his appetite.

• • • • • •

WEEK BY WEEK CHANGES FOR A HEALTHIER DIET

It is important to make any changes to your diet gradually. Aim to make a couple of changes a week. If you are still finding it hard to adjust to the initial changes allow yourself longer to get used to them before making any more. Below are some suggestions you might like to try.

WEEK 1
- Change from white to wholemeal bread.
- Try grilling instead of frying.

WEEK 2
- Replace a sugar snack with fresh fruit.
- Switch from butter to a low fat spread.

WEEK 3
- Try baked beans which have no added salt or sugar.
- Change from whole milk to semi-skimmed.

WEEK 4
- Cut down on sugar by buying canned fruit in natural juice instead of syrup.
- Eat less red meat and more fish and poultry.

WEEK 5
- Change to a breakfast cereal high in fibre.
- Don't add salt when cooking.

WEEK 6
- Add more vegetables to the plate and cut down on the amount of red meat portions.
- Cut down on sugar in recipes and use some wholemeal flour in place of white.

Looking ahead to the future

With a predicted fall in school leavers available for employment in the 1990's more women will be encouraged to fill the gap in the employment market. At present about 31% of women with a child under the age of five go out to work. Many more women are returning to work relatively soon after the birth of their first baby. In the period between 1950 and 1954, 13% of women having their first baby returned to work within one year and 20% within 2 years. By the period 1970–1974, these figures had risen to 22% and 30% respectively. The most up-to-date figures for this particular trend show that nearly 50% of women who are working when they become pregnant, return to work within nine months of the birth of their baby.

RETURNING TO WORK

A woman does not always have a free and clear cut choice when it comes to deciding whether to return to work or stay at home full time. This may be due to financial pressures within the family. Another reason may be the fact that many women are having their first baby at an older age when they are more established in their career and may feel under pressure to return to work early for fear of losing their status if they have a prolonged period out of the workplace. For some women, it may be a very positive decision based on the clear realisation that staying at home full time is not for them.

Mothering involves caring and comforting, teaching and stimulating, feeding and clothing and generally taking care of your child's needs. It does not necessarily mean that you have to be by your child's side constantly 24 hours a day and 365 days a year. It is the quality of the time you spend together that is important rather than the quantity. Knowing this doesn't automatically make the decision to leave your child in someone else's care part of the time any easier.

Whether or not your decision to return to work is something you choose to do or something you feel you have no choice about, it is bound to be difficult at first to leave your child. Many women struggle with tremendous feelings of guilt at the possible effects of their actions on their child. Once the decision has been made, if you have done all you can to ensure that your childcare arrangements are as caring and consistent as possible for your child, then try not to let guilt spoil either the time you spend with her or the time you are away from her. Time spent feeling guilty really is time wasted.

Forward thinking and planning are the key to making your return to work as smooth as possible. Preparing the way long before the actual day helps to minimise any worries you may have although it is bound to take time for both of you to get used to the change in your situation.

Combining Breastfeeding and Working

You will need to decide what will suit you and your baby best and this will depend largely on the age of your baby and whether or not you are returning to work full time. If you can take maternity leave until your baby is four to six months old, you should find it much easier than leaving a very young baby who is fully breastfed. Most babies are on solid food by the age of six months and will probably take drinks from a cup which makes it a little easier when you leave them.

It is possible with good planning to successfully combine breastfeeding and working, but only you can decide on what will suit your circumstances. If you decide to wean your baby fully off the breast before you return to work, it does require time so don't leave it until the last minute.

Many mothers continue to partially breastfeed when working, by feeding the baby as late as possible in the morning before leaving for work and feeding the baby on their return and doing any night feeds that are required. The baby then has bottles of either expressed breastmilk or formula milk during the day. Most babies will cope perfectly well with a combination of breast and bottle in this way providing they have had time to get used to this system of feeding.

Whether you are returning to work full-time or part-time, you may choose to continue fully breastfeeding, leaving bottles of expressed breastmilk for the childminder to give during the day. You can build up a store of expressed breastmilk in the freezer over a period of weeks before you go to work. It will be much easier to express some milk to store once your milk supply is well established than in the very early days when you are building up your milk supply and getting used to feeding your baby.

Expressing breastmilk at work may be necessary for your own comfort and to produce sufficient for your baby's needs. Discuss with your employer in advance when and where you will express the milk and where you will keep it.

It is important to cool the milk quickly once collected and make sure that you don't add newly collected warm milk to the previous

batch. It is hard to express milk if you are in a rush so try after a bath or shower or try expressing the second breast straight after a feed. First thing in the morning may be the time you feel that you have most milk.

Some mothers find that storing milk in the compartments of a sterilised ice tray is particulary convenient, as they can then thaw a few ice cubes quickly. If you are expressing milk at work, you will need to be extra careful about hygiene and the storing, and also the transporting of your milk as germs multiply very readily in warm milk. Electric breastpumps, which make it easier to express the milk, can be hired through your local NCT branch. For more information see the NCT leaflet *How to express and store breastmilk*.

Get your baby used to taking a bottle long before you leave her for the first time. It is probably worth introducing her to sucking from a teat, perhaps by giving boiled water initially, some time before you intend to go back to work. It will seem strange to her at first if she has always been totally breastfed and it might be a good idea for someone other than you to give her the bottle. If she smells your lovely familiar scent which she associates with snuggling up to your breast for a feed, she is unlikely to be really interested in the bottle. She will also need to become familiar with the person who is going to be looking after her. Having a short trial run of leaving her with that person for very short periods initially might be helpful in putting your mind at rest. See the NCT leaflet *Breastfeeding–Returning to work*.

It will be a matter of trial and error until you sort out what is right for the two of you. The most important thing is to keep calm about it all. If you get panicky and anxious that she is going to starve when you leave her because she will not take a bottle, it is going to take all the longer for you both to get settled. Many mothers find that their baby steadfastly refuses to take the bottle from her but happily accepts it from others.

Childcare Arrangements

This is an area of prime concern and one that is not easy to organise. There are a number of different options to choose from and finding the right one for you may take some time. If there is a working mums group within your local NCT branch do get in touch, you will find it extremely helpful to talk to other mothers who have already trodden this path and discovered some of the pitfalls. It also means that you can maintain that important contact with other mothers even though you are out at work all day.

The Working Mothers' Association has useful information packs and booklets and a book to help you sort your way through the maze of different options.

You or your partner may have the opportunity to share the care, or you may be lucky enough to have a family member close by who is willing to look after her.

Childminders provide the solution for many mothers. Childminders are people who look after children under five-years-of-age in their own home. They should be registered by the local authority who will have checked that the premises are safe for young children and followed up references. One of the advantages of having a childminder is that it gives your child the chance to play with other small children. One disadvantage is that if your child is ill you may not be able to take her to the childminder's in case she passes on any infection to the other children.

A nanny or mother's help will usually live in with the family, although they may come in on a daily basis. You could probably find one through local contacts or by putting an advertisement in magazines such as *The Lady* or *Nursery World*. The Working Mothers' Association has a very useful booklet which sets out all the information you might need about interviewing nannies, getting references, conditions of service and tax and national insurance etc.

It may be possible to share a nanny or come to some mutual childcare arrangement or job-share with another mother who also requires someone to look after her child. Alternatively, a nursery run by the Local Authority may be the answer. For details about these nurseries, contact the local council and if possible speak to other mothers who have used one.

One of the biggest difficulties any mother has to face is the tiredness and pressure on her time. It is vital to sort out with your partner, areas of responsibility regarding childcare and household tasks. The first step is to look realistically at how much time each task takes. The next step is to set some boundaries about making time for each other, and recognise the importance to you as an individual and to your relationship with your family of occasionally having some time to yourself. Feeling constantly worn out and resentful about all aspects of your life is no joke for anyone.

Organisation will be the key to juggling your time. The mornings are likely to be particularly stressed if you have to get the baby up, fed and dressed and off to the childminders in a rush in order to catch a train or bus, to say nothing of getting yourself ready

> **66** *Don't make the first day you go back to work the first time you leave the baby.*
>
> *The first day was awful. I thought about her all day, wondering if she was alright. I found that she had been and after that I was okay.* **99**

as well. Help to ease the situation by organising as much as you can the night before. Negotiating more flexible working hours with your employer, so that you can avoid rush hour travel, may help ease the pressure considerably.

You may have decided, after a period at home with your young baby that you want to return to paid work but would like to try something new rather than returning to your old job. Even though you know it is the right thing for you, you may also feel a certain lack of confidence about launching into something totally new.

If you think about all the things you have been responsible for while successfully running a home and taking care of children, they all involve skills which can be transferred to the workplace. These days more and more people are coming to value the skills that a mother has. If you sit down and write out a list of what you do at home, you may well be surprised at just how many skills are needed as a mother and homemaker.

• Being responsible for the household budget requires financial skills.

• Organising the many and varied activities related to running a home and caring for a family requires organisational skills, as well as taking responsibility and decision making.

• Dealing with the day to day complicated relationships and keeping the peace calls for diplomacy and communication skills.

• Tackling a number of different tasks at the same time shows you are capable of flexibility, adaptability, reliability and working to deadlines.

Libraries and job centres will have information about positions available, as well as possible training courses. The Working Mothers' Association has a practical pack full of useful information for women returning to work. There are other useful addresses at the end of this chapter.

LOOKING AFTER YOURSELF

The information in this book is aimed mainly at helping you to get in shape in the first few months following the birth of your baby.

In the coming months and years, your life will frequently change. You may have more children, elderly parents may become more dependent upon you, you may return to work or take on new interests and hobbies. Through all these changes and the demands made upon you, there will be a need to look after yourself as a woman in your own right and not just because so many others are dependent upon you.

In 1984, the Women's National Commission (WNC) set up a working party to study the provisions made for women by the National Health Service and to look at those health areas of greatest relevance to women. One of the findings of this study was that the level of care which postnatal women received was often inadequate and a number of the women questioned about their care said they would have greatly valued the opportunity to attend informal postnatal groups or classes.

For many years the NCT has been addressing that need by organising informal postnatal get togethers where women can meet others in similar circumstances. The Trust is now training postnatal exercise teachers who will work in conjunction with trained group leaders to offer exercise and discussion classes to postnatal women. At the time of writing, there are only a few branches which offer these particular classes but the situation will improve as more and more teachers are trained. If you are interested, do contact your local branch for further details.

Another finding of the WNC report related to preventive care and showed that there was a good deal of regional variation in the interpretation of the concept of Well Woman Centres and in the provision of such clinics or centres. These clinics or centres were meant to take a positive attitude towards women's health and provide a full check-up service for women. The original plan was that they should be for women, staffed by women and should attract all women and not just those who were ill, pregnant or seeking contraceptive advice. The idea was that they should encourage women to take responsibility for maintaining good health, provide self-help groups and counselling for people suffering from things like pre-menstrual or menopausal problems, sexual problems and addiction to smoking and alcohol.

In the WNC survey, 42% of those questioned did not know whether there was a Well Woman centre in their area and yet most Health Authorities questioned replied that they had made some provision for Well Women centres. If these facilities are available for women, why don't the women they are intended to help know about them?

Do you have such a centre in your area?
If so, what does it offer you?
If not, why not?

You could begin by asking your local Community Health Council what they provide for the health needs of the women in your area. In many areas the family planning clinic is called a well woman clinic but does not offer the wide range of facilities mentioned above. It is very likely that women who do not need or want information about contraception, will not attend these centres at all. Many women said they were too shy to visit the GP's surgery for some of the problems mentioned, particularly if the GP was a man. In a study in Manchester, two thirds of the women attending the well woman clinic were found to have an untreated medical problem.

We have a right to information and advice about our health, to expect that it is given to us in the most appropriate way. Most health

care policy makers and budget managers are men, with no real understanding of the specific problems which many women have. While this is the case we are unlikely to get the full and adequate provision we deserve. The only way to bring about any change is to keep on asking for the things we need.

No matter how busy your life, don't neglect your own health. Make sure that you have regular cervical smear tests. This test can detect pre-cancer cells in the cervix (neck of the womb) before cancer develops. Early detection and treatment greatly improves the cure rate. You will have a cervical smear at your postnatal check-up and you should then have one every 3–5 years. Keep a note of the date and if you do not receive a call-up from the GP when your next smear is due, you should ask for one.

Breast cancer is the commonest form of cancer in women but if detected early enough treatment has a very good chance of success. Once you stop breastfeeding, you should carry out self examination of your breasts each month. There is a useful leaflet available from the Health Education Authority or your GP which will show you exactly how to examine your breasts correctly. You will gradually become familiar with the way your breasts feel. If you then detect any significant changes in their look or feel, such as puckering or lumps, you should arrange to see your doctor as soon as possible. Most lumps turn out to be perfectly harmless but it is best to make sure. If there is a problem, any delay will only increase the risks to your health.

Mammography is a type of X-ray which shows up very early changes in breast tissue. It is normally advised for women over the age of 50 unless you have a particular problem which needs further investigating or if you have a history of breast cancer in your family.

Smoking is a major source of ill-health and death in this country and the longer you smoke the greater the risk to your health.

Unfortunately the numbers of young women who smoke are on the increase. The good news is that you can dramatically reduce any risk to your health as soon as you stop smoking. You may have given up or at least cut down on the amount you smoked during your pregnancy. If you have stopped, don't be tempted to start again.

If you have managed to cut down, it is worth trying to give up altogether. Babies whose parents smoke are more at risk of respiratory infections, so you would be doing yourself and your family a favour if you could manage to give up. It won't be easy but there are a few tips which might help you to achieve your goal. Knowing why you smoke is the first step towards helping you to stop. Keep a diary for a week and jot down all the times you had a cigarette, what was happening at the time and how you felt i.e.

- Do you use cigarettes as a confidence booster?
- Do you use cigarettes to help you concentrate?
- Do you use them to help you cope with stressful situations?
- Is it simply habit that makes you light up everytime you have a drink or a cup of tea or after a meal?

Once you have identified when and why you smoke, you can plan to do something else at a time when you would usually have a cigarette or learn to relax in some other way.

Many people worry that giving up smoking will make them fat. This is not inevitable and shouldn't really be a reason for not giving up. Smoking is a far greater risk factor than being overweight. The average weight gain caused by the effects on the metabolism of giving up the smoking, is only likely to be about 1.8–2.3 kg (4–5 lb). People often eat to compensate for not being able to smoke and if they eat high fat and sugar type snacks that will cause the weight gain. Be positive about giving up smoking.

- Think of the benefits to your health and also to your pocket.
- Choose a time when you are not under too much stress. Pick a day to STOP.
- Think of yourself as a non-smoker from the start. Sit in non-smoking areas and if someone offers you a cigarette say 'No thanks, I don't smoke' rather than 'I'm trying to give up.'
- Take one day at a time.

Remember you won't be alone, millions of others have given up successfully. If you experience side effects, the first few weeks are likely to be the worst and you may feel awful, but it will pass. The cravings will get less over the weeks and you will gradually feel fitter.

GOOD HEALTH

Good health is about improved quality of life in all its dimensions – physical, mental and social. It is not merely about avoiding illness.

Much of the responsibility for good health lies with us as individuals. By making some positive changes in your lifestyle, you will not only influence your own health and well-being but also that of your family. The early weeks and months of motherhood may be a time of renewed or newly awakened body awareness when you may come to recognise how much better you feel through taking appropriate and enjoyable exercise.

It is likely to be a time when you find yourself taking stock of many of the values and attitudes you have held for many years. It may be a time of personal growth and developing relationships as well as a time for learning many new skills.

Recognising the importance of having a healthy body and a healthy lifestyle should go a long way to preventing problems in later life. By recognising the importance of retaining independence and self-responsibility you are likley to find your self-esteem improved and the ability to enjoy motherhood as well as the other dimensions of your life greatly increased.

IDEAS FROM OTHER MOTHERS

I was delighted when the NCT decided to do exercise classes, it was an important turning point in feeling fitter and gave me a guideline that I was not as unfit as I thought. I enjoyed the postnatal classes and I was spurred on to more energetic classes.

. . . . . .

It is likely to be a time when you find yourself taking stock of many of the values and attitudes you have held for many years. It may be a time of personal growth and developing relationships as well as a time for learning many new skills.

. . . . . .

I feel as if I've now joined the club – my mother can now talk to me about everything.

. . . . . .

My mother loves her as much as I do, we've got something in common, we can talk together and I know I'm not boring her.

. . . . . .

Recognising the importance of having a healthy body and a healthy lifestyle should go a long way to preventing problems in later life. By recognising the importance of retaining independence and self-responsibility you are likely to find your self-esteem improved and the ability to enjoy motherhood as well as the other dimensions of your life greatly increased.

. . . . . .

I'd be stricter and ask people not to visit so early. I don't think anyone, except perhaps your mother should be there for the first couple of weeks. It's difficult to have lots of relatives especially if they expect to be fed.

Try and get dressed if you can.

. . . . . .

I didn't want to use a dummy but it's great now.

. . . . . .

Prepare and freeze in advance or buy ready-prepared meals.

. . . . . .

It takes such a long time to get ready to go out. Have a bag of all the baby gear you might need, ready and packed.

. . . . . .

I'd try giving a bottle earlier – it would have been so nice to get out a bit more.

. . . . . .

I had a portable TV in the bedroom – even if I didn't get dressed, I could keep up to date.

. . . . . .

One piece of good advice I was given is to enjoy each day with my baby as it comes. Older mothers and my own mother pointed out that it is so easy to spend time wishing that your baby could smile, sit up, walk, talk etc. that you forget to enjoy them as they are now and only later realise that you have spent some of their best times, which are so fleeting, wishing your baby would grow up quickly. This really helped me in the early days when I felt very tired and my son seemed so unresponsive.

. . . . . .

I think talking to other women who had had babies was helpful in preparing me for the arrival of my baby. However it struck me afterwards that no one had told me about the really good parts.

USEFUL ADDRESSES

The National Childbirth Trust (NCT),
Alexandra House,
Oldham Terrace,
Acton,
London W3 6NH
Tel: 081-992 8637

(The National Childbirth Trust is Britain's best-known charity concerned with education for parenthood. It is run by, and for, parents through its network of 350 branches and groups. It offers information and support in pregnancy, childbirth and early parenthood and aims to enable every parent to make informed choices.)

NCT (Maternity Sales) Ltd.,
Burnfield Avenue,
Glasgow G46 7TL
Tel: 041–633 5552

Association of Chartered Physiotherapists in Obstetrics and Gynaecology,
11, Bayview Road,
Aberdeen AB2 6BY

Association of Breastfeeding Mothers,
26, Holmshaw Close,
London SE26 4TH
Tel: 081-778 4769

Association for Postnatal Illness,
25, Jerdan Place,
Fulham,
London SW6 1BE
Tel: 071-386 0868

Breakthrough Trust (Organisation run by deaf people for deaf people),
Charles Gillette Centre,
Selly Oak Colleges,
Bristol Road,
Birmingham B29 6LE
Tel: 021-472 6447

British Sports Association for the Disabled,
34, Osnaburgh Street,
London NW1 3ND
Tel: 071-383 7277

Caesarean Support Network,
2, Hurst Park Drive,
Huyton,
Liverpool L36 1TF
Tel: 051-480 1184

Child Poverty Action Group,
1–5 Bath Street,
London EC1
Tel: 071-253 3406

Disabled Living Foundation,
380–384 Harrow Road,
London W9 2HU
Tel: 071-289 6111

Family Planning Association,
27–35 Mortimer Street,
London W1N 7RJ
Tel: 071-636 7866

Gingerbread (for single parents),
35, Wellington Street,
London WC2E 7BN
Tel: 071-240 0953

GLAD (Greater London Association for the Disabled),
336 Brixton Road,
London SW9 7AA
Tel: 071-274 0107

A range of childcare leaflets for blind mothers are available in Braille and on cassette from:
Yvonne Rowe,
Heathersett College,
Philanthropic Road,
Redhill,
Surrey RH1 4YZ
Tel: 0737 768935

Health Education Authority,
Hamilton House,
Mabledon Place,
London WC1H 9TX
Tel: 071-383 3833

INTERHEART
(Aims to put people in touch with others who suffer from similar heart conditions)
The Chest, Heart and Stroke Association,
Tavistock House North,
Tavistock Square,
London WC1
Tel: 071-490 7999

Kids Club Network,
Oxford House,
Derbyshire Street,
London E2 6HG
Tel: 071-247 3009

La Leche League,
BM3424,
London WC1N 3XX
Tel: 071-242 1278

Look After your Heart: Look After Yourself,
Project Centre,
Christ Church College,
Canterbury,
Kent CT1 1QU
Tel: 0227 455687
(Trains tutors who run LAY classes for the general public, which include safe individual exercise and relaxation programmes and group discussions on health topics such as healthy eating, stress, alcohol and smoking.)

Mary Marlborough Lodge (A residential assessment centre to help disabled parents adjust to life with a new baby)
Nuffield Orthopaedic Centre,
Headington,
Oxford OX3 7LD
Tel: 0865 64811

MIND (National Association for Mental Health),
22, Harley Street,
London W1N 2ED
Tel: 071-637 0741

NAWCH (National Association for the Welfare of Children in Hospital),
Argyle House,
29–31 Euston Road,
London NW1 2SD
Tel: 071-833 2041

National Childminding Association,
8, Masons Hill,
Bromley,
Kent BR2 9EY
Tel: 081-464 6164

National Council for One Parent Families,
235, Kentish Town Road,
London NW5 2LX
Tel: 071-267 1361

Parentline,
Rayfa House,
57 Hart Road,
Thundersley,
Essex SS7 3PD
Tel: 0268 757077

Pre-School Playgroups Association,
61–63 Kings Cross,
London WC1X 9LL
Tel: 071–833 0991

REMAP
25, Mortimer Street,
London W1N 8AB
Tel: 071-637 5400

Royal National Institute for the Blind,
224–228 Great Portland Street,
London W1V 6AA
Tel: 071-388 1266

Royal National Institute for the Deaf,
135A High Street,
Acton,
London W3 6LY
Tel: 081-993 4748 (voice)
Text: 081-993 4691 (300 Baud)

Spinal Injuries Association,
76 St James' Lane,
London N10 3DF
Tel: 081-444 2121

Women Returners Network,
Euston House,
81–103 Euston Street,
London NW1 2ET
Tel: 071-388 3111

Working Mothers Association,
77 Holloway Road,
London N7 8JZ
Tel: 071-700 5771

Working for Childcare,
77 Holloway Road,
London N7 8JZ
Tel: 071-700 0281
(Promotes research and development and
information on work related childcare)

YMCA London Central Training and
Development Department,
112, Great Russell Street,
London WC1B 3NQ
Tel: 071-580 2989
(Offers specialist training in Antenatal and
Postnatal Exercise to RSA qualified exercise
and music teachers)

SUGGESTED FURTHER READING

Ann Dickson (1982): *A woman in your own right. Assertiveness and you.* Quartet books.

Ann Oakley (1974): *The Sociology of Housework.* Martin Robertson.

Melanie Henwood, Lesley Rimmer and Malcolm Wicks (1987): *Inside the Family. Changing roles of men and women.* Family policy studies centre.

Mukti Jane Campion (1990): *The Baby Challenge.* Tavistock/Routledge.

Rodney Cullum and Lesley Mowbray (1986): *The English YMCA Guide to Exercise to Music.* Pelham books.

Sheila Kitzinger (1989): *Breastfeeding your baby.* Dorling Kindersley.

Richard Seel (1987): *The Uncertain Father.* Gateway Publications, Bath.

SUGGESTED MUSIC

Warm-up and cool-down sections:

I will survive
Gloria Gaynor
The look of love
ABC

Build-up aerobics:
I should be so lucky
Kylie Minogue
Together forever
Rick Astley
You and I
Fleetwood Mac

Hard aerobic section:
Rush hour
Jane Wieldlin
Hooked on classics (Scotland the Brave)
Louis Clark conducting the R.P.O.

MSE section:
You Win Again
Bee Gees
The Girl is Mine
Michael Jackson and Paul McCartney
Listen to your heart
Roxette

Stretch section
It would take a strong strong man
Rick Astley
Your song
Elton John
Coming in and out of your life
Barbra Streisand

REFERENCES

1. MacArthur C, Lewis M, Knox EG and Crawford JS (1990) *'Epidural Anaesthesia and long term backache after childbirth'.* BMJ vol 301, 7 July 1990 pp 9–12.

2. Rutherford O. (1990) *'The Role of exercise in prevention of Osteoporosis'.* Physiotherapy Sept 1990 Vol 76 no 9. pp 522–526.

3. Henwood M, Rimmer L and Wicks M. (1987) *'Inside the Family: Changing roles of men and women'.* Family Policy Studies Centre Occasional paper.

Index